Assessing the Need for a Comprehensive National Health System in the United States

Nikolaos Karagiannis
Winston-Salem State University, USA

Sheilia R. Goodwin
Winston-Salem State University, USA

David Stewart
Winston-Salem State University, USA

A volume in the Advances in Healthcare Information Systems and Administration (AHISA) Book Series

IGI Global
PUBLISHER of TIMELY KNOWLEDGE

Published in the United States of America by
IGI Global
Information Science Reference (an imprint of IGI Global)
701 E. Chocolate Avenue
Hershey PA, USA 17033
Tel: 717-533-8845
Fax: 717-533-8661
E-mail: cust@igi-global.com
Web site: http://www.igi-global.com

Library of Congress Cataloging-in-Publication Data

Names: Karagiannis, Nikolaos, 1964- editor. | Goodwin, Sheilia Rae, 1948- editor. | Stewart, D. B., editor.
Title: Assessing the need for a comprehensive national health system in the United States / Nikolaos Karagiannis, Sheilia Rae Goodwin, and David Bruce Stewart, editors.
Description: Hershey, PA : Information Science Reference, [2023] | Includes bibliographical references and index. | Summary: "This multidisciplinary edited book examines at theoretical and, especially, policy levels, a number of key aspects related to the U.S. health system, presenting different perspectives, providing facts and data-based assessments and offering alternative strategies, policies, and realistic options towards a better and healthier U.S. society"-- Provided by publisher.
Identifiers: LCCN 2021052232 (print) | LCCN 2021052233 (ebook) | ISBN 9781668440605 (hardcover) | ISBN 9781668440612 (paperback) | ISBN 9781668440629 (ebook)
Subjects: LCSH: Medical care--Evaluation--Methodology. | Medical care--Evaluation--United States. | Public health--United States.
Classification: LCC RA399.A1 A876 2022 (print) | LCC RA399.A1 (ebook) | DDC 362.10973--dc23/eng/20211220
LC record available at https://lccn.loc.gov/2021052232
LC ebook record available at https://lccn.loc.gov/2021052233

This book is published in the IGI Global book series Advances in Healthcare Information Systems and Administration (AHISA) (ISSN: 2328-1243; eISSN: 2328-126X)

British Cataloguing in Publication Data
A Cataloguing in Publication record for this book is available from the British Library.

All work contributed to this book is new, previously-unpublished material.
The views expressed in this book are those of the authors, but not necessarily of the publisher.

For electronic access to this publication, please contact: eresources@igi-global.com.

Advances in Healthcare Information Systems and Administration (AHISA) Book Series

Anastasius Moumtzoglou
Hellenic Society for Quality & Safety in Healthcare and P. & A. Kyriakou Children's Hospital, Greece

ISSN:2328-1243
EISSN:2328-126X

MISSION

The **Advances in Healthcare Information Systems and Administration (AHISA) Book Series** aims to provide a channel for international researchers to progress the field of study on technology and its implications on healthcare and health information systems. With the growing focus on healthcare and the importance of enhancing this industry to tend to the expanding population, the book series seeks to accelerate the awareness of technological advancements of health information systems and expand awareness and implementation.

Driven by advancing technologies and their clinical applications, the emerging field of health information systems and informatics is still searching for coherent directing frameworks to advance health care and clinical practices and research. Conducting research in these areas is both promising and challenging due to a host of factors, including rapidly evolving technologies and their application complexity. At the same time, organizational issues, including technology adoption, diffusion and acceptance as well as cost benefits and cost effectiveness of advancing health information systems and informatics applications as innovative forms of investment in healthcare are gaining attention as well. **AHISA** addresses these concepts and critical issues.

COVERAGE

- Measurements and Impact of HISA on Public and Social Policy
- Virtual health technologies
- Management of Emerging Health Care Technologies
- IT Applications in Health Organizations and Practices
- IS in Healthcare
- Clinical Decision Support Design, Development and Implementation
- Decision Support Systems
- E-Health and M-Health
- Role of informatics specialists
- Telemedicine

IGI Global is currently accepting manuscripts for publication within this series. To submit a proposal for a volume in this series, please contact our Acquisition Editors at Acquisitions@igi-global.com or visit: http://www.igi-global.com/publish/.

Titles in this Series

For a list of additional titles in this series, please visit: http://www.igi-global.com/book-series/

Digital Identity in the New Era of Personalized Medicine
Ingrid Vasiliu-Feltes (University of Miami, USA) and Indira Mysore (Bloqcube Inc., USA)
Medical Information Science Reference • © 2023 • 315pp • H/C (ISBN: 9781799889663) • US $325.00

Advanced Bioinspiration Methods for Healthcare Standards, Policies, and Reform
Hadj Ahmed Bouarara (Dr. Moulay Tahar University, Algeria)
Medical Information Science Reference • © 2023 • 325pp • H/C (ISBN: 9781668456569) • US $295.00

Cases on Lean Thinking Applications in Unconventional Systems
Eduardo Guilherme Satolo (São Paulo State University, Brazil) and Robisom Damasceno Calado (Fluminense Federal University, Brazil)
Engineering Science Reference • © 2023 • 262pp • H/C (ISBN: 9781668451854) • US $240.00

Handbook of Research on Complexities, Management, and Governance in Healthcare
Ubaldo Comite (University "Giustino Fortunato" Benevento, Italy)
Medical Information Science Reference • © 2023 • 411pp • H/C (ISBN: 9781668460443) • US $470.00

Revolutionizing Healthcare Through Artificial Intelligence and Internet of Things Applications
Keshav Kaushik (University of Petroleum and Energy Studies, India) Susheela Dahiya (University of Petroleum and Energy Studies, India) Ashutosh Dhar Dwivedi (Copenhagen Business School, Denmark) and Shilpi Aggarwal (State University of New York, USA)
Medical Information Science Reference • © 2023 • 330pp • H/C (ISBN: 9781668454220) • US $345.00

IGI Global
PUBLISHER of TIMELY KNOWLEDGE

701 East Chocolate Avenue, Hershey, PA 17033, USA
Tel: 717-533-8845 x100 • Fax: 717-533-8661
E-Mail: cust@igi-global.com • www.igi-global.com

Table of Contents

Section 2
Technological and Human Capital Challenges

Section 3
Cultural and Institutional Attributes

Detailed Table of Contents

Following World War II, European governments embarked on high levels of social spending and expanded the welfare state. Part of the explanation for the post-war welfare state development in the continent lies with the impact that the war itself had on European society. The destruction was so massive that it generated new social needs and created new demands among citizens. The presence of strong labor movements and socialist and left-wing parties also played a key role in the expansion of the European welfare state given their emphasis in the protection and promotion of social rights. Indeed, most European constitutions following the Second World War were influenced by socialist parties. But the situation was quite different on the other side of the Atlantic, and this chapter explains some of the reasons for the failure of the US to develop a European-style welfare state.

There are different systems of government and different beliefs worldwide. Some countries have governments that are highly involved in the healthcare of their populations, with national healthcare systems that offer universal coverage for all citizens. Other countries have governments that allow the private sector to control the majority of the healthcare industry. Considering that both options have positive and negative aspects, this chapter presents both pros and cons of government-controlled healthcare.

This chapter first provides the two main theoretical perspectives related to the U.S. health system: the "market-based" view and the "socially sensitive" argument. The second main section discusses important facts and highlights related to the national health situation of the United States compared with other advanced OECD countries. Taking these facts and highlights into consideration, the final sections of the contribution critically examine the merits and demerits of contrasting approaches to implementing a comprehensive national health and insurance scheme in the United States, and offer concrete policy considerations. Some brief conclusions end the chapter.

This chapter describes the difference between health and health care, the efficacy and efficiency of the US health care system, the institutional framework of the US healthcare system, and the positive and negative features of the system, as well as recommendations for change. The authors note that US healthcare is both among the world's best and the developed world's worst, depending on what is being used as a basis for comparison. The complexity of the system with its seven different methods of payment is taken to task, and the fact that health care is an industry that significantly deviates from classical economic industrial theory is evaluated in depth. It is noted that economics can tell us much about how the misaligned and inappropriate incentives, as well as the erroneous comparisons to other industries, have allowed politicians to mislead the public as to the true benefits and drawbacks of the US health care system, which is better described as "sick care" as opposed to "health care."

Section 2
Technological and Human Capital Challenges

The U.S. government and its population incurs more out-of-pocket expenses in terms of per capita than ever before. The question that arises as a result is: does the increased expenditure result in either improved quality or quicker access to healthcare? To answer this question, the role modern technology plays in the deliverance of healthcare is analyzed in this chapter. An important conclusion that can be drawn from this analysis is that the U.S. needs to fund research to develop, monitor, and implement healthcare technologies that will allow physicians to supplement and improve their practices. Further, capacity management of beds and increased investment into healthcare in general appears to be critical, regardless of how effectively technology is used.

This chapter examines the utilization of telehealth from its inception to the recent prodigious increase in utilization during the Covid-19 pandemic. Delivery methods, including synchronous and asynchronous methods as well as remote and mobile health, are described. Its history and utilization in rural and exceptional settings and its comparative efficacy with traditional care are reviewed. Legal questions, including those related to autonomy, confidentiality, licensing, and jurisdictional concerns are presented. Finally, trends and a review of the prospects for the future of telehealth are examined.

This chapter discusses the current state of healthcare workers in the United States and strategies that show promise in mitigating shortages. Although some strategies involve leveraging technology, it is more important to provide students with an

Preface

Setting the Context

There is significant debate regarding the quality of the national health system of the United States relative to those of other countries. The U.S. healthcare system has been heavily criticized as a highly inefficient, disorganized, fragmented, and under-resourced primary care system that contributes to high healthcare costs, high rates of uninsured individuals, and a number of health problems in comparison to the situation in other Western nations. What's more, the United States is currently the only wealthy industrialized country that has not achieved universal health coverage. Together, these reasons help explain why important health indicators have been deteriorating during the last years. For example, the U.S. life expectancy has, for the first time since the 1960s, gone down during the past five years or more.

Yet, most countries worldwide use single-payer systems to cover all their citizens. According to different national and international sources (e.g., the Commonwealth Fund, Health Systems Facts, the U.S. Census Bureau, WHO, OECD), during the last 20 years, the best countries for healthcare are the United Kingdom, the Netherlands and Australia, with the United States being consistently the lowest performer among the developed countries. In fact, the United Kingdom ranked first, and the other countries in the comparison were Australia, Switzerland, Sweden, the Netherlands, New Zealand, Norway, Germany, Canada, and France. The United States fared poorly on such important measures as affordability, access, health outcomes, and equality between the rich and poor. Not surprisingly, the rate of uninsured Americans varies by race, ethnicity, and social group.

Consequently, the healthcare reform debate in the United States has been an intense political topic focusing upon increasing medical coverage, decreasing costs, insurance reform, in addition to the philosophy of its provision, funding, and government involvement. As medicine in the United States is big business, and as the health and insurance sectors have been frequently paying significant amounts of money to House and Senate members –with Lawmakers that chair key committees being leading recipients–, much of the debate has involved how the different sides are competing to express their views, rather than the specific reform proposals.

U.S. health policy has been consumed by an ideological divide between conservative and liberal viewpoints. Conservatives, on the one hand, point to freedom of choice and regard the passage of healthcare reform as "a precarious path towards Europeanization of the United States", with the Federal Government becoming more intrusive.[1] Liberals, on the other, have long been the primary advocates for both Social Security and Medicare, which are often pursued as significant government policies that have overwhelming satisfaction of basic social needs. According to their argument, healthcare is a fundamental human right, which is based on Article 25 of the *Universal Declaration of Human Rights*: "Everyone has the right to a standard of living adequate for the health and well-being of himself and of his family, including food, clothing, housing and medical care and necessary social services".[2] Similarly, Franklin D. Roosevelt argued that the *Bill of Rights* had proved inadequate to assure Americans equality in the pursuit of happiness, and advocated for a right to medical care in his 1944 proposal for a *Second Bill of Rights*.[3]

Undoubtedly, the disjointed U.S. healthcare looks like it has been on the verge of transformation for years, if not decades. The current coronavirus contagion has stressed healthcare systems around the world, testing their capacities to care for patients and protect health workers in a time of crisis. In the United States, in a matter of few months, the coronavirus pandemic has exacerbated ongoing challenges and has revealed deep long-standing drawbacks of its health system, which have accelerated digital health choices at a pace few could have imagined. Contemporary healthcare demands have contained the seeds of a wider critique of the American health system, leading social movements and political campaigners to adopt calls for universal coverage across the country. Implementing a comprehensive single-payer health system and achieving health equity will be the toughest policy challenges that will require uncomfortable changes for them to become real.

ORGANIZATION OF THE BOOK

The multidisciplinary edited book *Assessing the Need for a Comprehensive National Health System in the United States* seeks to thoroughly examine at theoretical and, especially, policy levels a number of key aspects related to the U.S. health system. With important contributions by distinguished academics and professionals, the book seeks to present different perspectives, provide a facts and data-driven assessment, and offer alternative strategies, policies, and realistic options towards a better and healthier U.S. society.

This edited volume is structured around three main themes, which are also the titles of the three sections of the book. Section, titled "Economic and Public Policy Considerations", contains Chapters 1-4. In the opening chapter, Karagiannis and Polychroniou discuss several controversial theoretical issues related to the social responsibilities of government. The authors then analyze some broad but important public policy areas and challenges, and offer policy considerations that could help the United States to address its social development and welfare shortcomings.

In Chapter 2, Foster and Goodwin claim that there are different systems of government and different beliefs worldwide. According to the authors, some countries have governments that are highly involved in the health, illness, and healthcare of their populations with national healthcare systems that offer universal coverage for all citizens whereas other countries have governments that allow the private sector to control the majority of the healthcare industry. Considering that both options have positive and negative aspects, the chapter presents both pros and cons of government-controlled healthcare.

In Chapter 3, Stewart, Goodwin and Karagiannis provide main theoretical perspectives related to adopting a comprehensive national health system in the United States, and discuss important facts and highlights related to the country's overall health situation compared with other advanced OECD countries. Taking these facts and highlights into consideration, the authors critically examine the merits and demerits of implementing a comprehensive national health system in the United States, and offer concrete policy considerations.

In Chapter 4, Madjd-Sadjadi and Marcelli discuss the difference between health and healthcare as these are often misunderstood concepts in discussion of the efficacy and efficiency of the U.S. healthcare system. The authors then examine positive features of the healthcare system of the United States and lay down its institutional framework. Finally, the chapter assesses drawbacks and offers concrete recommendations for changes to the current system in the United States.

Section 2, titled "Technological and Human Capital Challenges", comprises Chapters 5-8. Chapter 5 by Karagiannis, Gosavi and Gosavi argues that effective technological progress can be a significant contributing factor to an improved health system in the United States. According to the authors, the United States needs to fund research to develop, monitor, and implement healthcare technology and generate healthcare policy that will benefit the citizens and allow physicians to supplement and improve their practices. The successful implementation of healthcare technology in a variety of different medical settings will allow for a better healthcare system in the United States.

Chapter 6 by Joseph and Greene focuses on challenges and prospects associated with telehealth and telemedicine in rural healthcare delivery. According to the authors, although telemedicine use in the U.S. has increased over the past several years, it was primarily used to reach those in rural areas who traditionally faced multiple barriers to accessing consistent, quality healthcare. Joseph and Greene further contend that the changing face of telehealth may contribute to increased health disparities in the United States, which may be exacerbated by unresolved legal questions and great inconsistency in the laws and regulations, from state to state.

Chapter 7 by Harp discusses the shortage of various types of healthcare workers in the United States by focussing on the numbers of healthcare professionals needed, and provides strategies that show promise in mitigating shortages. Diversity and inclusion efforts along with the important role of historically black colleges and universities (HBCUs) to addressing the country's shortage of healthcare workers are also included in the author's analysis.

In Chapter 8, Liu aims to advocate for pharmacists' provider status on the federal level. To achieve this status, the author specifies three main objectives: 1. to describe the background and efforts for pharmacists to obtain provider status; 2. to demonstrate the benefits of the expanded pharmacy practice scope using two selected pharmacy services; and 3. to discuss the future of pharmacy practice. According to Liu, pharmacists also need to educate the public, other healthcare professionals, third party payers, policymakers, and legislators about why obtaining provider status is imperative.

Section 3, titled "Cultural and Institutional Attributes", consists of Chapters 9-11. Chapter 9 by Scriven unpacks and lays bare three stories which demonstrate how education, healthcare, and social justice are necessary ingredients of a 3-sided pyramid. These stories – which have African Americans in the Deep South and health insurance at the center– demonstrate that without the unifying foundation of neighbor love, deep education, true healing, and abiding social justice can never be achieved. According to the author, these stories are profoundly universal in that they reflect shared aspiration, suffering, striving, and inevitable triumph.

In Chapter 10, Foster argues that, out of 195 countries in the world, the United States is one of the few developed countries that does not offer free, universal healthcare for its citizens. The United States is also one of the countries with the highest debt, and a large portion of this debt can be contributed to healthcare spending. According to the author's line of argument, although the U.S. healthcare system exhibits many positive qualities, it has a lot of room for improvement and advancement.

In the last chapter of the book, Tepepa argues that although the United States government passed legislation and stabilization packages to respond to the COVID-19, especially in 2020 and 2021, the response to the global pandemic has been hindered by the lassitude of the state and the prevailing conception of social policy that leaves the most vulnerable unprotected. In addition to the systemic obstacles, the access to healthcare by noncitizens faces changes to immigration law that penalize recipients of certain social services on grounds that they are a public charge, which further restricted their access to treatment and hindered the fight against the pandemic.

Our task would have been incomplete if we had not acknowledged all those who kindly aided us in completing this edited volume. We would like to thank the distinguished contributors for their willingness to participate and respond to our suggestions, and the advisors and staff of IGI Global who have provided excellent support throughout the preparation of this manuscript. We would also like to thank the *Journal of Best Practices in Health Professions Diversity: Research, Education, and Policy* and the Levy Economics Institute of Bard College for kindly permitting versions of the essay "Does the United States Need a National Health and Insurance Scheme? Views, Facts, Challenges, and Potential Benefits" (first published in *J Best Pract Health Prof Divers*, Vol. 13, No. 2, Fall 2020) and the Working Paper No. 950 (April 2020) to appear as chapters 3 and 11 respectively in this edited volume. We would like to acknowledge valuable research assistance by Vasileios T. Karagiannis and Charalampos A. Karagiannis in areas of public policy and finance. Last, but not the least, we would like to thank our families for their continuous support and encouragement, and our colleagues and students for their inducements. We owe them more than we can recount.

Nikolaos Karagiannis
Winston-Salem State University, USA

Sheilia R. Goodwin
Winston-Salem State University, USA

David Stewart
Winston-Salem State University, USA

ENDNOTES

1 Charlie Rose-Senator Judd Gregg interview, March 2010. Archived from the original on September 13, 2012.

2 The Universal Declaration of Human Rights is an international document adopted by the United Nations General Assembly that enshrines the rights and freedoms of all human beings. It was accepted by the General Assembly as Resolution 217 during its third session on December 10, 1948 in Paris, France.

3 During his Eleventh State of the Union Address on Tuesday, January 11, 1944.

Section 1
Economic and Public Policy Considerations

Chapter 1
Addressing the Social Policy and Welfare Deficit of the United States:
Key Notions and Policy Implications

Nikolaos Karagiannis
Winston-Salem State University, USA

C. J. Polychroniou
Independent Researcher, USA

ABSTRACT

Following World War II, European governments embarked on high levels of social spending and expanded the welfare state. Part of the explanation for the post-war welfare state development in the continent lies with the impact that the war itself had on European society. The destruction was so massive that it generated new social needs and created new demands among citizens. The presence of strong labor movements and socialist and left-wing parties also played a key role in the expansion of the European welfare state given their emphasis in the protection and promotion of social rights. Indeed, most European constitutions following the Second World War were influenced by socialist parties. But the situation was quite different on the other side of the Atlantic, and this chapter explains some of the reasons for the failure of the US to develop a European-style welfare state.

DOI: 10.4018/978-1-6684-4060-5.ch001

INTRODUCTION: THE CONTEXT

Following World War II, European governments embarked on high levels of social spending and expanded the welfare state. Part of the explanation for the post-war welfare state development in the continent lies with the impact that the war itself had on European society. The destruction was so massive that it generated new social needs and created new demands among citizens, according to Obinger and Schmitt (2017). The presence of strong labor movements and socialist and left-wing parties also played a key role in the expansion of the European welfare state given their emphasis in the protection and promotion of social rights. Indeed, most European constitutions following the Second World War were influenced by socialist parties. Accordingly, by the 1950s, a consensus had emerged between conservative and social democratic/socialist parties throughout Western Europe on the principles of the postwar socio-economic order. The capitalist market would be regulated, while the state would guarantee the provision of free social services, such as, healthcare and education at all levels, social housing and generous benefits.

Although costly, the welfare state was perceived by most European governments as a 'social investment' that can bring about multiple tangible and intangible benefits and would pay itself along the way. The expansion of the welfare state depended on taxation and expenditures incurred for redistributive or growth purposes. In almost all western European states, the most important reason for the increase in the government expenditure/GDP ratio was government transfers to households due to demographic changes and the advent of social security programs. The more general cause of the rapid growth of transfer payments was the increasing demand for 'merit' goods (e.g., education, health, social security) in most European countries. Clearly, the welfare arrangements are more developed in some countries than in others, and the nature of government involvement is also different among different countries. However, in general, since the 1980s, the attempt to control government spending by setting ceilings on budget deficits has resulted in a decreasing expansionary effect of public expenditures (OECD, n.d.).

Social programs in the United States are programs designed to ensure that the basic needs of the American population are met. There are federal and state social programs which include health insurance, cash assistance, food assistance, housing subsidies, energy and utilities subsidies, and education and childcare assistance. Similar benefits are sometimes provided by the private sector either through policy mandates or on a voluntary basis. In fact, the American government sector has played an important role in the development of these private plans. Employer-sponsored health insurance is an example of this. American social programs vary in eligibility with some, such as public schooling, are available to all while others, like housing subsidies, are available only to segments of the population. Programs are offered by various organizations on a federal, state, local, and private level. This diversity in services and service populations helps to provide for basic needs like food, shelter, education, and healthcare to residents of the U.S. through primary and secondary education, subsidies of higher education, pensions, health insurance programs, unemployment and disability insurance, subsidies for eligible low-wage workers, subsidies for housing, and Supplemental Nutrition Assistance Program benefits. Social Security, Medicare and Medicaid are the country's prominent social programs (Wikipedia.org, "Social programs in the United States").

Historically, the United States has been spending less on social policies and welfare programs compared with advanced European countries, in terms of gross public social welfare expenditure. Such social welfare spending varies between different states in the U.S. The country tends to tax lower-income people at lower rates, and relies substantially on private social welfare programs and philanthropy. Since the late 19th century, notable government initiatives to promote social welfare took place:

- During the late 19th and early 20th centuries, attempts were made to move poor people who were seeking relief funds from work yards to "poor houses." Colonial legislatures and later State governments adopted legislation patterned after the English "poor laws". By 1929, workers' compensation laws were in effect in all but four states.
- From 1890 to the early 1920s, according to Skocpol (1995), the U.S. offered 'maternalist policies' which provided pensions for widowed mothers. This was the first large-scale social policy program in the United States that sought to support the Civil War veterans and their families and provide pensions and disability assistance. Aid to veterans, often free grants of land, and pensions for widows and handicapped veterans, have been offered in all U.S. wars. Following World War I, provisions were made for a full-scale system of hospital and medical care benefits for veterans.
- Prior to the *Great Depression*, the United States had social programs that mostly centered around individual efforts, family efforts, church charities, business workers compensation, life insurance, and sick leave programs along with some state tax supported social programs. The misery and poverty of the great depression threatened to overwhelm all these programs. The severe Depression of the 1930s made Federal action necessary as neither the States and the local communities, businesses and industries, nor private charities had the financial resources to cope with the growing needs among the American people. Beginning in 1932, the Federal Government first made loans, then grants, to states to pay for direct relief and work relief. After that, special Federal emergency relief and other public works programs were started.

- Franklin D. Roosevelt argued that the *Bill of Rights* had proved inadequate to assure Americans equality in the pursuit of happiness. The *Social Security Act of 1935* was signed into law by Roosevelt, created the Social Security program as well as insurance against unemployment, and was part of his New Deal domestic program.
- In 1940, *Aid to Families with Dependent Children* (AFDC) was established by the Social Security Act of 1935 as a grant program to enable states to provide cash welfare payments for needy children who had been deprived of parental support or care because their father or mother was absent from the home, incapacitated, deceased, or unemployed. All 50 states, the District of Columbia, Guam, Puerto Rico, and the U.S. Virgin Islands operated an AFDC program.
- In the 1960s, *War on Poverty* was an expansive social welfare legislation that was introduced by the administration of Lyndon B. Johnson and was intended to help end poverty in the United States. It was part of a larger legislative reform program, known as the "Great Society," that Johnson hoped would make the United States a more equitable and just country.
- In 1996, the *Personal Responsibility and Work Opportunity Reconciliation Act* passed under Bill Clinton and became law. The law was a cornerstone of the Republican Party's "Contract with America" and also fulfilled Clinton's campaign to "end welfare as we know it." Yet, by signing the 1996 Act, President Clinton "made the biggest reactionary shift in social policy since the Great Depression" and "essentially put an end to welfare as an entitlement program" (Polychroniou, 2021).
- In 2010, the *Affordable Care Act* (ACA), formally known as the *Patient Protection and Affordable Care Act,* and colloquially known as *Obamacare*, is a United States federal statute that was signed into law by Barack Obama. Both the Affordable Care Act and the Health Care and Education Reconciliation Act of 2010 represent the U.S. system's most significant regulatory overhaul and expansion of healthcare coverage since the enactment of the Medicare and Medicaid programs in 1965 (Wikipedia.org, "Social programs in the United States").

Clearly, the acceptance of socioeconomic inequality, and the limited development of government programs in the areas of welfare and healthcare are quite evident in the United States. This adverse development is contrary to Article 25 of the *Universal Declaration of Human Rights* which states that "Everyone has the right to a standard of living adequate for the health and well-being of himself and of his family, including food, clothing, housing, and medical care and necessary social services" (The Universal Declaration of Human Rights is an international document adopted by the United Nations General Assembly that enshrines the rights and freedoms of all human beings. The document was accepted by the General Assembly as *Resolution* 217 during its third session on December 10, 1948 in Paris, France). Veto points in the U.S. structure of government make social programs in the country resilient to fundamental change. As of 2020, the public social spending-to-GDP ratio in the United States was below the OECD average. In other words, "politics explains why the United States did not develop a European-style welfare state. Political factors also explain why economic inequalities are so huge in the US and the middle class is shrinking; why the quality of America's healthcare system is dead last when compared with other western, industrialized nations; why there are millions of homeless people; and why the infrastructure resembles that of a third-world country" (Polychroniou, 2021).

With this background in mind, the subsequent main sections discuss controversial theoretical issues related to the social responsibilities of government, and analyze some broad but nevertheless important public policy areas and challenges that could help the United States to address its social development and welfare shortcomings. Brief conclusions end the chapter.

CONTROVERSIAL THEORETICAL ISSUES

The majority of macroeconomic policies are related to, and influenced by, fiscal policies. Indeed, the world economy is often subject to large changes in fiscal policies. Until the mid-1970s, governments tended not to run deficits (OECD, n.d.); but since the early 1980s, a lot of criticism has been directed against Keynesian economic policies, which were seen as the intellectual basis that provided the green light for governments to intervene excessively and to run budget deficits. 'New Right', economic neoliberalism, and Washington Consensus perspectives were underpinned by strong anti-government beliefs, and attempted to limit the scope of state activity by denying any possibility of alleviating social problems and ills by means of policy intervention. The large size of the government sector was argued to be detrimental to the growth prospects of the economy and directly responsible for inflation. Privatisation of state activities was hailed as the modern miracle 'antidote' to various economic 'ills.' Legislation was often employed by governments in order to decrease the public expenditure and, especially, the social welfare payments (Karagiannis and Madjd-Sadjadi, 2007).

Since the 1980s, the dimensions of economic policies pursued by a number of governments of developed economies (in the U.S., the U.K., and elsewhere), were largely dictated by the intellectual force of such arguments: large-scale privatisations, the abandonment of the commitment to full employment, the reduction of public sector employment, substantial reforms in industrial relations legislation and a number of other similar measures were presented as a means of reducing the frontiers of the state. "The tendency by political administrations to accept the principle of a more limited role of the state has had the effect of arresting the growth of government expenditure as a ratio of GDP" (Hadjimatheou, 1994, p. 322).

Looking at the OECD data (n.d.), it is noticeable that many countries have reduced their education and health budgets, and there has clearly been a considerable reduction in the rate of growth of expenditure on education and health services in relation to GDP. Critics of the reforms sometimes point out that the massive decrease of people on the welfare rolls during the 1990s wasn't due to a rise in actual gainful employment in this population, but rather, was due almost exclusively to their offloading into 'workfare' giving them a different classification than classic welfare recipient. The late 1990s were also considered an unusually strong economic time, and critics voiced their concern about what would happen in an economic downturn. As Barr (1992, p. 795) points out, "despite the new ideology, neither the Thatcher (and the Major) nor the Reagan administrations actually succeeded in rolling back the boundaries of the Welfare State."

Since the beginning of the 1980s, national fiscal policies have exhibited large divergences, and all the major countries (the USA, the UK, Germany, France, and Japan) have followed a relatively contractionary course. Fiscal policy tightened in Europe over the same period, and this was, in general, the trend since the 1980s. All these "are connected to the nature of the political spectrum that exists in Europe and, more specifically, to the European social [welfare] model with its emphasis on social protection, pensions, public services, workers' rights, quality of jobs, working conditions, and environmental concerns, even though [...] the social [welfare] model has been under attack since the early 1980s and has certainly been weakened as a result of European Union policies promoting market efficiencies, liberalization and competition law, privatization, and financialization" (Polychroniou, 2021). Differences in public spending vary widely between countries. It is noticeable that in most countries the rise in public spending continued until the early 1980s; but since then, public expenditures levelled off or started to decline as a share of GDP while slow economic growth added new burdens on the budget (Karagiannis and Madjd-Sadjadi, 2007).

For most countries, the last decades have been characterised by an increase in the share of public debt in GDP, as well as periods of important increases in real interest rates, two factors which contribute to increasing the debt payment. At present, fiscal policy in Europe is still tight, providing no economic stimulus to growth and higher levels of employment. Looking at the IMF data (*World Economic Outlook*, various years), high and volatile real rates of interest, large fluctuations in real exchange rates, and significant variations in private sector spending are also noticeable. The co-movements of GDP growth rates and the main fiscal variables (government expenditure and tax revenue) reflected the outcomes of macroeconomic policies as well as unexpected shocks and world happenings. Changes in the main fiscal variables and the induced changes in GDP were associated with corresponding adjustments of private sector spending, namely, consumption and investment. These policies, which were undertaken by the major economies, affected the rest of the World (Karagiannis and Madjd-Sadjadi, 2007).

Clearly, during the last 40 years, the appearance of 'big' governments, without a corresponding increase in tax revenues, along with efforts to finance government deficits, has shifted the emphasis of policy towards financial control and away from government expenditure planning. At least during the last two decades or so, frequent economic crises seem to have seriously affected attitudes towards government expenditure and, as a result of the recent pandemic, most governments have been forced to redirect their policy priorities. The recent global plague has important implications for adjustment policies which governments have followed in order to maintain a 'reasonable balance' between economic adjustments and social welfare.

With respect to the U.S. welfare programs, in particular, the American social security system is considered by many observers to be seriously flawed and inadequate. As Polychroniou (2021) has remarked,

The American welfare state is organized around different principles –it functions primarily around tax expenditures and public-private partnerships– than the welfare state in other advanced nations, thanks to the dominance of conservative modes of thinking with regard to the relationship between individual and society (partly due to the influence of the Protestant work ethic which looked with suspicion of anyone who is poor, and partly due to free-market economics which rejected outright the role of the government in promoting overall social well-being), but also due to the uniqueness of American federalism.

When not reciting bogus arguments about [budget] deficits and debt in connection with increased federal spending, [conservative and right-wing politicians and commentators] have always opposed every new social program targeted on the poor and average Americans on purely ideological grounds. For them, the welfare state leads inevitably to socialism (and, for the grandfather of neoliberalism, F. A. Hayek, to totalitarianism), but naturally they keep silent about the massive government support that the corporate and financial industries receive when their fortunes turn sour. So, it's ok to offer socialism to the rich. But for everyone else, brutal capitalism should be the order of the day (Polychroniou, op. cit.).

Some of the key issues include sustainability, the impact of the system on economic growth, and the equity of the system for various participants. The U.S. social security system is a 'pay-as-you-go' scheme, meaning that payroll taxes on today's workers and employers pay for the current social security benefits of retired workers. But the sustainability of the system can become an issue when the ratio of retirees to workers becomes too large to finance. With the aging of the 'baby boomer' generation, policy makers are concerned about the long-term financial viability of the currently structured social security system. For the free marketers, the option of private investment accounts would establish personal retirement accounts, managed by private pension and investment companies, with part of the social security tax currently paid by workers.

Private investment accounts make America's social security system more of a 'public-private partnership.' Proponents of this policy proposal state the potential for a higher rate of return on retirement savings, thereby addressing the sustainability issue. Opponents of this policy option point out the lack of egalitarianism, and warn of the market risks and relatively high administrative costs of private investment accounts. The fundamental problem is the conflict between the goals of quality of life and cost containment, especially when minimizing costs takes priority over the coverage of basic social needs and overall welfare. Such considerations historically have provided service with an emphasis on social needs in contrast to other criteria such as ability-to-pay or profit.

ADDRESSING THE CHALLENGES

The economic effects of the continuous financial crises and the current pandemic are complicated and far-reaching because of simultaneous shocks in the stock, housing, and labor markets. Actual spending, job creation, home equity, well-being, emotional and physical health, and expectations about the future have all been affected by these calamities. What's more, there are various political, institutional, and cultural challenges related to American social welfare, especially those concerning the development of policies and programs that will better address major social problems and issues in the United States. Egalitarian solutions cannot rely on philanthropy that serves to diminish social displeasure with the high rate of inequality that is present in American society. The common thinking is manifested in two main ways: "first, wealth in America, in general, has not been passed down for so many generations that people look at it as 'unearned''' and, second, "the wealthy often act to bring themselves into greater esteem through philanthropic endeavors while paying reduced tax obligations" (Harwell, Karagiannis and Madjd-Sadjadi, 2013, p. 119).

All these problems are in principle solvable but require genuine and purposeful interventions with teeth. And executive policy makers need to 'circle back' and consider alternative realistic policy options. First, fiscal policy along 'functional finance' lines can secure funding for necessary social programs that have a positive impact on economic growth and income distribution in the United States (Lerner, 1943). The 'functional finance' approach would argue whether budget deficits and government debt that are too large ought to be judged against the 'functional finance' benchmark, and would place special emphasis on the roles of fiscal policies in supporting selected egalitarian social welfare plans.

Secondly, a different public finance outlook is vital in the United States. European governments, "regardless of whether they are using the Nordic or the Christian-Democratic socioeconomic model, have far more generous social programs than those provided by the US government." Accordingly, total spending on "social protection benefits in the EU is equivalent to approximately 27 percent of GDP, while in the U.S. it is just over 18 percent of GDP, and they reach a significantly larger share of citizens" (Polychroniou, 2021). In a similar vein, Wade asserts that "[a government that performs the necessary welfare functions] has a level of taxation (perhaps supplemented by aid) sufficient to provide public expenditure on physical infrastructure, education and health, significantly higher than in economies following the liberal market model, [...] equivalent to at least 35 percent of GDP" (2014, pp. 3-4). Accordingly, as the Federal receipts have always been less than 20 percent of GDP (for detailed statistical information, see U.S. Office of Management and Budget (OMB), various years), precisely due to an erroneous narrative about how the business sector serves as the sole wealth creator, the U.S. taxation system and legislation would need significant changes in order to effectively address tax avoidance and loopholes.

What Keynes argued in *How to Pay for the War* (1940) is relevant here. Reducing inequality and effectively addressing tax avoidance and loopholes would require a different public finance outlook that emphasizes the fundamental principles of 'social justice' and 'ability-to-pay.' Given that about 47-51 percent of federal revenue comes from individual income taxes, around 6-11 percent from corporate income taxes, and another 33-35 percent from payroll taxes that fund social insurance programs (Tax Policy Center, 2021; Office of Management and Budget, various fiscal years), such a view clearly assumes that raising taxes on rich Americans and large corporations would make a more fair and meaningful contribution to the public good.

Adopting the crucial social sensitivity for a better and more humane U.S. society, as European governments do, the U.S. federal government would spend considerably more on unemployment insurance, and should engage in more direct regulations in order to protect working people against business interests. Unsurprisingly therefore, even in the age of global neoliberalism, where social programs are under constant attack, the welfare state remains an ideal that most European and other advanced societies appreciate regardless of partisanship (for instance, the National Health System in Great Britain).

However, "none of the above is meant to convey the idea that the U.S. should necessarily try to imitate the European social [welfare] model. At this historical juncture, the U.S. should be leaning forward into a path of [sustained] economic development, [significant social welfare advancement], social justice, and environmental sustainability" (Polychroniou, 2021). These notions are truly bold policy considerations to addressing the well due social policy and welfare deficit in the United States. They also help molding alternative policies and ideological stance of 'unorthodox' political groups and people while refuting negative and meaningless terms and views used by highly reactionary and conservative forces of the U.S. political and social spectrum.

CONCLUSION

This chapter leaves many vexing problems unsolved. Much detailed planning would be needed to facilitate further development of social welfare policies in the United States. Social, racial, linguistic, geographic, and other nonfinancial barriers to access would persist. Establishing comprehensive policy priorities and masterfully directing funds to high-quality investigations would be of paramount importance. Further work in long-term areas would be required. Regional planning and capital allocation would enable, but not ensure, the fair and efficient allocation of resources. Finally, although all these problems would not be solved, a technically proficient national welfare program would establish a framework for addressing them.

Assuming that modern policy interventions ought to be socially sensitive and egalitarian, we propose a realistic framework for public debate on fundamental policy requirements. Many of the largest corporations would enjoy substantial cost savings if such a proposal were adopted. More significantly, the great majority of Americans would greatly benefit from a comprehensive, publicly administered welfare program. If mobilized, such public conviction could override even the most strenuous private and political opposition. A sophisticated understanding of the need for socially sensitive government action is requisite to appropriate selection of thorough, technically proficient, and well-planned welfare strategies and policies.

REFERENCES

Barr, N. (1992, June). Economic Theory and the Welfare State: A Survey and Interpretation. *Journal of Economic Literature, 30*(2), 741–803.

Hadjimatheou, G. (1994). In P. Arestis & M. Sawyer (Eds.), *"Public Expenditure," in The Elgar Companion to Radical Political Economy* (pp. 319–323). Edward Elgar.

Harwell, G. A., Karagiannis, N., & Madjd-Sadjadi, Z. (2013). A Production-oriented Strategy for the United States: A Framework of Alternative Developmentalist Notions. In N. Karagiannis, Z. Madjd-Sadjadi, & S. Sen (Eds.), *The US Economy and Neoliberalism: Alternative Strategies and Policies* (pp. 115–143). Routledge.

IMF, World Economic Outlook, Washington, DC: IMF, various issues.

Jansson, B. S. (2001). The Reluctant Welfare State: American Social Welfare Policies-Past, Present, and Future (4th ed., pp. 194, 199). Wadsworth/Thomson Learning.

Karagiannis, N., & Madjd-Sadjadi, Z. (2007). *Modern State Intervention in the Era of Globalisation.* Edward Elgar.

Keynes, J. M. (1940). *How to Pay for the War: A Radical Plan for the Chancellor of the Exchequer*. Macmillan.

Lerner, A. P. (1943, February). Functional Finance and the Federal Debt. *Social Research, 10*(1), 38–51.

Marx, J. D. (1997). Federated Fundraising. In *The International Encyclopedia of Public Policy and Administration* (Vol. 2, pp. 877–881). Westview Press.

Obinger, H., & Schmitt, K. (2018, May). The Impact of the Second World War on Postwar Social Spending. *European Journal of Political Research, 57*(2), 496–517. doi:10.1111/1475-6765.12236

OECD, (n.d.). *National Accounts,* (vol. II). OECD. https://www.oecd-ilibrary.org/economics/national-accounts-of-oecd-countries-volume-ii-detailed-tables_19961995

Palley, T. I. (1998, Fall). The Economics of Social Security: An Old Keynesian Perspective. *Journal of Post Keynesian Economics, 21*(1), 94. doi:10.1080/01603477.1998.11490181

Polychroniou, C. J. (2021). So-called Democratic 'Moderates' Are Actually Right-wingers Who Have Always Thrown up Roadblocks to Social Progress. *Common Dreams*. https://www.commondreams.org/views/2021/09/14/so-called-democratic-moderates-are-actually-right-wingers-who-have-always-thrown

Post, J. E., Lawrence, A. T., & Weber, J. (2002). *Business And Society: Corporate Strategy, Public Policy, Ethics* (10th ed.). McGraw-Hill.

Skocpol, T. (1995). Protecting Soldiers and Mothers: The Political Origins Of Social Policy. In *The United States* (pp. 290–293). Harvard University.

Social Programs in the United States. (n.d.). In *Wikipedia*. https://en.wikipedia.org/wiki/Social_programs_in_the_United_States

Tax Policy Center. (2021). *What Are the Sources of Revenue for the Federal Government*. Urban Institute and Brookings Institution. https://www.taxpolicycenter.org/briefing-book/what-are-sources-revenue-federal-government

Trattner, W. I. (1999). From Poor Law To Welfare State: A History Of Social Welfare. In *America* (6th ed., p. 348). The Free Press.

Wade, R. H. (2014). The Developmental State: New Perspectives. JICA/IPD Task Force Meeting on Industrial Policy & Transformation, Jordan, June 5-6.

Chapter 2
The Role of Government in National Healthcare Systems:
A Global Perspective of Pros and Cons

Melissa Robin Bowman Foster
Winston-Salem State University, USA

Sheilia R. Goodwin
Winston-Salem State University, USA

ABSTRACT

There are different systems of government and different beliefs worldwide. Some countries have governments that are highly involved in the healthcare of their populations, with national healthcare systems that offer universal coverage for all citizens. Other countries have governments that allow the private sector to control the majority of the healthcare industry. Considering that both options have positive and negative aspects, this chapter presents both pros and cons of government-controlled healthcare.

INTRODUCTION

Throughout history, governments around the world evolved to meet the needs of people. Since the earliest days of mankind, cultures around the world have endeavored to understand the meanings of health and illness and to discover practices to maintain health or prevent illness. With different systems of government and different beliefs, nations must determine the extent of involvement of government in health and illness, what services will be available, to whom services will be available, and how the

DOI: 10.4018/978-1-6684-4060-5.ch002

services will be funded, offered, and monitored for quality. Some countries have governments that are highly involved in the health, illness, and healthcare of their populations with national healthcare systems that offer universal coverage for all citizens. Other countries have governments that allow the private sector to control the majority of the healthcare industry (Straube, 2012). Both options have positive and negative aspects, and it is up to each country to determine how large, or small, of a role the government will have in the healthcare system. This chapter will present both pros and cons of government-controlled healthcare.

GOVERNMENT-CONTROLLED HEALTHCARE: PROS

In this section, the positive aspects to government-controlled healthcare will be discussed. Examples will be provided from countries that currently use a high level of intervention, or control, on the healthcare system and have positive outcomes for citizens as well as the healthcare system. Many countries with government-controlled healthcare believe that access to healthcare is a human right and that it is the responsibility of the society and government to assure this right. In 1948, the United States (US) and 47 other countries signed the United Nations Universal Declaration of Human Rights which stated that, "everyone has the right to a standard of living adequate for the health and well-being of oneself and one's family including [...] medical care" (WHO, 1978). The US and other members of the WHO met in 2005 to sign World Health Assembly resolution 58.33 stating that everyone should have access to healthcare services and should not have financial hardship (WHO, 2013). The US is currently the only one of 38 countries who belong to the Organization for Economic Cooperation and Development (OECD) that does not have government-controlled healthcare. The idea of government-controlled healthcare has been a politically divisive topic, especially since the passing of the Affordable Care Act in 2010. There have been attempts to extend Medicare and Medicaid, most recently during the 2016 election period –nicknamed, "Medicare for all." The bill was sponsored by US Senator Bernie Sanders, who wrote:

Healthcare must be recognized as a right, not a privilege. Every man, woman, and child in our country should be able to access the healthcare they need regardless of their income... We need a system that works not just for millionaires and billionaires, but for all of us. Americans should not have to fear losing their health insurance if they lose their job or change employment... We need a system that prioritizes the health of working-class families over the profits of insurance companies.

Therefore, proponents of government-controlled healthcare see healthcare as an internationally recognized right (Fisher, 2022; Kelly, 2010; Sanders, 2017;WHO, 1978). They advocate to decrease the number of uninsured, lessen the financial burdens people face paying for healthcare, and expand or extend eligibility for existing coverage and shifting the costs to the federal government (Sanders, 2017; Thorpe, 2016). Some proponents focus on people who are currently uninsured or face particularly high healthcare spending burdens (Curtis et al., 2022; Dao & Mulligan, 2016; Friedman, 2021); others support a more inclusive program similar to Medicare and Medicaid that would provide healthcare to all Americans through a federal, government-controlled healthcare program (Fisher, 2016; Fox & Poirier, 2018; McGrath et al., 2022; Wang, 2021).

Protection from Health-Related Discrimination

A common practice shown by numerous private health insurance companies in the past is the refusal of coverage, or only offering limited coverage, based on a person's pre-existing medical conditions. People who are suffering from diabetes, heart disease, chronic illnesses such as sickle cell anemia, cystic fibrosis, and other conditions have historically been at risk of being refused medical coverage by insurance companies because of these pre-existing conditions. This prevented these people from freely looking for new and/or different insurance coverage because they knew the chances were high that they would be denied. For those who were using a group insurance plan through their employer, it sometimes limited them from changing jobs and/or working on their own business because they knew they would not be able to find decent health insurance coverage because of their pre-existing conditions. One group of people greatly affected was pregnant women, who would not be able to change jobs during pregnancy because there was a high chance their pregnancy, being a pre-existing condition, would result in them being refused medical insurance coverage, therefore they would lose health insurance coverage for the care needed during the remainder of their pregnancy, delivery, and post pregnancy (Huguet et al., 2019).

Government intervention allows regulations to be created and enforced to prevent insurance companies from using pre-existing conditions as reasoning for denying coverage. The regulations prevent insurance companies from discriminating against those who may be suffering from chronic illness.

Improved Population Health: Everyone is Covered

According to a report conducted and shared by the Centers for Disease Control, in 2020, there were 31.6 million people uninsured in the United States. Most people who do not have medical insurance will avoid seeking medical care unless it becomes extremely necessary. Most uninsured people do not receive preventive services due to the high out of pocket costs, which means there is a lower chance of early detection of medical conditions. Without early detection, many conditions will advance until signs and symptoms are more obvious and unbearable for the patient. When patients reach this point and finally do seek medical care, most diseases have advanced to more severe stages which requires more invasive, uncomfortable, and costly treatment (Parker et al., 2020).

With government-controlled healthcare, all citizens receive health insurance coverage. Health insurance coverage, in most cases, covers the full cost or majority of the cost for preventive services. Knowing services are covered and the out-of-pocket cost will be minimal motivates most people to seek preventive medical services. Preventive medical services allow for earlier detection of illness as well as continued monitoring of more chronic conditions to maintain health and ensure quality of life. This will help improve the health of the overall population and potentially lead to lower spending on more costly medical diagnosis (Galvani et al., 2020).

For example, the national health service in Italy is known as Servizio Sanitario Nazionale (SSN) and offers lab services, medications, primary care services, public hospital treatment, and some specialist care to Italian citizens for free or minimal cost. Since enacting this program in July 1980, research has shown a vast increase in Italian citizens now receiving preventive care services. Additionally, the number of chronic conditions diagnosed at later stages also decreased once the SSN was enacted and all citizens were eligible for medical coverage (Turati, 2013).

One of the major arguments against government-controlled healthcare in the US is that instituting government-controlled healthcare in the US will lead to socialism. Medicare, Medicaid, CHIP, and most recently the ACA are programs that provide government-controlled healthcare, but only to certain populations (Niles, 2015; Truglio-Londrigan & Lewenson, 2011). Medicare and Medicaid have been around for more than 50 years, and they have not led the United States to socialism. CHIP was signed into law in 1997 –25 years ago– and CHIP has not led the United States to socialism (Walker, 2015). To say that government-controlled healthcare leads to socialism is confusing association with causation (Parascandola, 1996). Although some countries with government-controlled healthcare may be socialist, not all socialist countries have government-controlled healthcare and not all countries with government-controlled healthcare are socialist. Given the long history of the US as a country which values individualism and independence, it is not likely that the US would be led to socialism by instituting government-controlled healthcare.

Accountability for Quality Health Services

Government intervention in healthcare can assist with ensuring top quality health services by assigning accountability to providers and healthcare organizations. Federal agencies can monitor the quality of health services being provided and create standards that must be met by medical practices. This, to some extent, has already been practiced in the United States by the Agency for Healthcare Research and Quality (AHRQ). The AHRQ focuses on improving the performance of health systems to ensure quality and safety for patients and healthcare professionals. The United States Department of Health & Human Services (HHS) is another area of the government that assists with offering a variety of health services and conducting health related research. With government involvement in nationwide healthcare, measures can be taken to set standards that will ensure quality care such as certification, accreditation, and licensure requirements that must be met for a medical practice to continue business and/or for a medical care provider to continue practicing. The federal government can also assist when problems are detected with the quality of medical care provided. When compromised care becomes an ongoing problem, government intervention can provide the necessary data collection and analysis to determine the root cause or causes of the problem and then provide assistance to resolve the issues (Chansatitporn & Pobkeeree, 2020).

Government agencies can also be used to address more specific issues in healthcare, such as the implementation of new technologies. For example, in Ireland the Health Information and Quality Authority (HIQA) is an agency funded by the Irish government which monitors healthcare quality. Within HIQA, another group has been established to ensure the proper implementation of electronic health records (EHRs) and the proper practice of maintaining those records and confidential information. The HIQA creates and implements standards that all medical practices in Ireland must follow to continue providing care to Irish citizens (McGrath et al., 2022).

Another concern with healthcare services is accessibility and waiting time for care. Again, this is something that can be regulated by government intervention. In Sweden, the Vardgaranti standard was established to ensure minimal wait times for medical services. The Vardgaranti has established a waiting time of seven days or less for primary care physician visits and a waiting time of 90 days or less for care from a specialist. If the wait will be more than 90 days, an agreement must be signed by both the physician and patient explaining why and when the care will be provided (Lapidus, 2017).

Possibility 1: Simpler, More Affordable Payments

Currently, the way payments are made for medical services can be overly complex for patients leading to a lot of confusion. Since the majority of American citizens use private insurance companies, they must be knowledgeable of the terminology to determine which plan is right for them. Each plan will have different components that will fall under the financial responsibility of the patient including the deductible, copay, and coinsurance. These are all in addition to the monthly surcharge patients pay to have coverage, known as the premium. Furthermore, patients will also need to be knowledgeable as to how different types of services are covered, or not covered, under each plan option. For example, many plans will have separate deductibles for outpatient and inpatient services. Many plans also have different copays based on whether the care provided was from a general practitioner or a specialist. Moreover, some plans may also charge extra fees for dental and vision coverage. When a patient finally receives the bill for medical services, they may be surprised to find out the services were not covered because of the type of plan they chose, the diagnostic codes did not justify the treatment codes, or that their financial responsibility is higher based on the type of care received requiring a higher deductible, copay, or coinsurance. It is common in the United States for privately insured people to receive high medical bills weeks or months after treatment (De Lew et al., 1992).

Germany is a country that has addressed this issue and eliminated this concern for German citizens. In Germany, a universal multi-player healthcare system has been implemented. Based on a person's salary, they will contribute to a statutory health insurance and/or private health insurance. The majority of healthcare services are paid for by employers and their employees, both contributing ~ 7-8% of the employees' salaries. For most medically necessary and preventive services, German citizens will not have any other out-of-pocket expenses. Most medications will cost German citizens between $0 - $11. For most scenarios, this has eliminated confusing medical bills for German citizens and unexpected out-of-pocket expenses (Altenstetter, 2003).

Possibility 2: Supporting Small Business Growth

Another potential result of the government providing universal healthcare to citizens is the support it would provide for small business growth. In 2020, studies showed that 54% of the United States population depended on employer-based health insurance. Due to the high cost of premiums for private plans offering sufficient coverage, many people depend on the group plans offered by their employers so they can pay a lower premium for coverage for themselves and their families. This need and dependency for lower cost health insurance has forced many citizens to choose working for a large corporation over the desire to start their own business. Small business owners usually are not able to offer health insurance coverage, so it is hard for them to find affordable coverage for themselves. Since they do not offer it as a company benefit, it can also be hard for them to find dedicated employees (Kwapisz, 2020).

With government sponsored healthcare for all citizens, the need to work for an employer who offers private group insurance is not necessary, allowing potential entrepreneurs more freedom to start their own business without having to worry about the necessity of health insurance. It would also help small businesses that cannot yet afford to offer a medical insurance benefit find employees since the medical insurance benefit would not be as high of a priority among potential hires.

ALLOWING MEDICAL PROFESSIONALS TO FOCUS ON PATIENT CARE

Due to the complexity of the United States healthcare system depending on payments from private insurance, some government sponsored insurance (Medicare, Medicaid, TRICARE, CHAMPVA), and self-pay patients, healthcare organizations are required to put a lot of time and resources into the accounts payable area. As confusing as different plans and their regulations are for the patients, this can be just as confusing and time consuming for the medical care providers. By simplifying this process and having a set amount that providers know they will receive for each patient, procedure, treatment, etc. it will eliminate much of the time needed for determining how much money will be received and from who for each patient bill. Additionally, in many cases healthcare organizations are also having to determine how much they will have to write off since different insurance companies and plans reimburse different amounts for specific procedures and the amounts may not cover the costs listed by the organization. (Chernew & Mintz, 2021). Simplifying the process by having all citizens on a universal healthcare plan that clearly communicates the amount that will be reimbursed for each procedure will eliminate the hours and resources needed for this work. This will allow healthcare organizations to dedicate more time and resources to patient care, possibly leading to improved care for patients and an improved work environment for employees.

GOVERNMENT-CONTROLLED HEALTHCARE: CONS

Opponents to government-controlled healthcare maintain that government-controlled healthcare is the antithesis of the culture of individualism, self-determination, and free enterprise that provides the basis for the healthcare system in the US (Niles, 2015). Opinions about government-controlled healthcare mirror attitudes concerning the government's role in general, and this is evident at any debates for healthcare reform (Blumberg & Holahan, 2019). The US healthcare system consists of a public sector and a private sector with some areas of the public sector being subsidized by the private sector. As with governmental function in general, the US has three governmental levels in the healthcare system –federal, state, and local– which have specific public health sector roles. There has historically been no centralized decision making in either the government or the healthcare system of the US (Aydin et al., 2021; Finkelman, 2015b).

The private sector provides most of the care to individuals in the US and includes healthcare services by profit and non-profit organizations and voluntary agencies with specific missions (Finkelman, 2015a; Montgomery, 2022; Walker, 2015; Wang, 2021). The public sector provides services for socially marginalized populations and reimburses private sector care to individuals through Medicare and Medicaid and the Children's Health Insurance Program (CHIP) (Finkelman, 2015b; Niles, 2015). Under the current system Americans are individually responsible for their own health and their own healthcare (Russia Today, 2010; Salsman, 2012).

Payment for healthcare services in the US is through a mix of out-of-pocket payments, health insurance plans, health savings accounts and government funding through Medicare, Medicaid, and CHIP. Most Americans access healthcare services through private insurance and health insurance is primarily accessed through employment (Statista Research Department, 2022). According to the Statista Research Department (2022), the majority of Americans have health insurance (92%) and about half of those who are insured receive private insurance through their employer, while an additional 34 percent are covered under the public insurance programs Medicare and Medicaid. More than 61% of employers provide health insurance coverage as a benefit for employees (Kaiser Family Foundation, 2012).

In discussion of pros and cons of government-controlled healthcare, most of the arguments can be grouped into three broad categories of costs, coverage, and values. These categories are not exhaustive, nor are they mutually exclusive. For example, discussion of healthcare workers can be included under either costs or coverage because anything that affects the healthcare workforce can at the same time increase or decrease both the costs of healthcare services and the ability to provide services (coverage). For heuristic purposes, issues affecting the healthcare workforce will be discussed under costs. While many people may consider costs as only monetary, costs also include people and services (Kambil, 2017; Nunn et al., 2020). Coverage may encompass whether or not individuals have access to services, how they get access to services—including healthcare insurance, how services are paid for and by whom, and what services are covered (Banthin, 2018; Finkelman,

2015a; Higgins Donius, 2011). Values covers belief systems, attitudes, and ethics (Aydin et al., 2021; Blumberg & Holahan, 2019; Niles, 2015; Walker, 2015). For each of the three broad categories, the cons of government-controlled healthcare are discussed in more detail in the sections that follow.

Costs

Costs are the major cause of controversy surrounding the topic of instituting government-controlled healthcare and financial or budgetary costs predominate discussions about costs (Kambil, 2017; Nunn et al., 2020; Sanders, 2017; Thorpe, 2016). However, the healthcare workforce (people) has become increasingly relevant in discussions about healthcare costs.

Financial or Budgetary Costs

The total amount spent on healthcare depends on the underlying cost of care. Overall costs of healthcare can be lowered by changing either the price or utilization of services. Government-controlled healthcare is attained through eliminating or reducing the private sector and growing the public sector to assume healthcare and healthcare costs for individuals. Government-controlled services are typically funded through increased taxes and/or increasing debt of the federal government leading to budget deficits. Promoters of government-controlled healthcare point to the high costs of healthcare in the US –$10,966 per capita in 2019 (Wang, 2021)– and claim that converting to a government-controlled system would lower healthcare costs. This ignores the fact that all change initiatives have costs and inadequate planning of the budget can set off a cascade of problems (Gregory, 2013; Kambil, 2017). Blahous (2018) projected that providing government-controlled healthcare to all American could increase federal spending by $32.6 trillion over the first 10 years of implementation. According to Kenneth Thorpe of Emory University, the plan for government-controlled healthcare introduced by Senator Bernie Sanders is underfunded by an average of almost $1.1 trillion per year. Holahan et al. (2016) estimated that government-controlled healthcare could actually increase federal spending by more than 50%. Shifting nearly all spending for healthcare from the private sector to the public section would require large increases in government spending (Blumberg & Holahan, 2019). The Committee for a Responsible Federal Budget calculated that switching to government-controlled healthcare would cause the federal debt to rise from 74 percent of GDP in 2015…to 154 percent of GDP by 2026. The cost of expanding coverage will be paid through higher taxes. According to Gregory (2013), funding a government controlled plan would cause payroll taxes to double, but Thorpe (2016) asserts that this change would require an even greater increase in payroll tax from 6.2% to 14.3%. The increase would be greater still for those earning over $250,000 per year—a 40% increase in income taxes (Thorpe, 2016). Thorpe adds that in addition to the impact on individual payroll taxes, small businesses would have a 6.2% payroll tax increase, while low income Medicaid recipients would pay a 2.2% income tax and a 6.2% income reduction. Government-controlled healthcare is paid through taxes and people who earn more would pay more taxes, subsidizing healthcare for those who earn less or are unemployed (Salsman, 2012). The US has already experienced persistently expanding administrative costs of Medicare and Medicaid (Diamond, 2009). Additionally, outcomes from states that have piloted government programs to expand access to care have ended in failure due to mismanagement, poor fiscal planning, and lack of foresight to expand the number of providers (Diamond, 2009; Draper et al., 2008; Friedman, 2021; Long, 2008; Myers, 2007).

The data on current government-controlled healthcare programs such as Medicare, Medicaid, and the Children's Health Insurance Program (CHIP) support the view that government-controlled healthcare programs produce "explosive growth" in spending and government debt (Ryan, 2011). All government programs that provide healthcare for certain segments of the population made up less than 10% of the federal budget in 1985 (Korobkin, 2014). By 2012, costs for the same programs made up 21% of the federal budget and if nothing changes, these costs are projected to be 30% of federal government spending by 2028 (Banthin, 2018; Korobkin, 2014). A study at George Mason University (Blahous, 2018) calculated that providing all Americans with the services currently received in Medicare, Medicaid, and CHIP would produce a growth in federal spending of more than 3 trillion dollars per year over the next 10 years.

The bottom line is that government-controlled healthcare would cost more than the current system in the US. Providing more coverage to more people may be a noble endeavor, but the fact is that healthcare needs to be considered in the "cold logic of dollars and cents, rather than the warm and fuzzy altruistic ideals;" thinking about healthcare as anything other than a commodity has to stop "before we run out of wallet" (McArdle, 2016).

People/Workforce Costs

In a review of the people costs for the healthcare workforce, the Hamilton Project (Nunn et al., 2020) noted that the healthcare sector employs slightly more than 10% of all workers in the US, but accounts for nearly 25% of government spending. A study of spending by non-hospital healthcare businesses put the cost of labor on average at almost 50% of their budgets. To lower labor costs, there needs to be an increased supply of labor or a change in the mix of who provides care and a reduction in unnecessary services (Nunn et al., 2020).

Healthcare Workers—Physicians and Nurses

Despite making up almost 10% of the US labor force (Nunn et al., 2020), the supply of healthcare workers has not been able to meet the demand or need. For physicians, one factor in shortages is that the profession limits the labor supply by limiting residency positions. According to Nunn et al. (2020), although there have been slight increases in residency positions, the number of residency positions continues to be lower than the number of applicants for residencies. The limitations on supply of physicians coupled with increased needs of an aging population has contributed to a shortage of physicians (Nunn et al., 2020). Doctor shortages in the US have led to a 30% increase in wait times (Heath, 2017). By 2030 there is projected to be a shortage of up to 104,900 doctors (Gudbranson et al., 2017). With a decrease in reimbursements for services and increase in practice restrictions predicted with the institution of a government-controlled healthcare system, the shortage is projected to be much worse.

Currently, salaries for managers who work for private insurers are much higher than salaries in the public sector for comparable positions (Friedman, 2021). In 2018, the head of the Centers for Medicare and Medicaid Services (CMS), in charge of coverage for a major portion of Americans, earned less than $250,000 while each of the CEOs of seven large health insurers earned over $16 million a year (Friedman, 2021). Government-controlled programs like Medicare and Medicaid also have to spend funds that could be used for salaries or services on policing eligibility of program participants. The CMS currently is able to leverage control of hospital pricing, drug pricing, and physician pricing. If a government-controlled healthcare system was instituted, hospitals, pharmacies, and physicians would be paid less for their services. Physicians in countries with government-controlled healthcare have incomes that range from 15 to 51% lower than US doctors (Book, 2009). For example, physicians in Britain and Canada have incomes more than 30 percent lower than their US counterparts (Book, 2009). If lower payments were established by a government-controlled healthcare system, by definition physicians could not drop out and make their living from other patients, because there wouldn't be any other patients. The only alternative for a physician would be to quit medicine and retire or find another profession. Many physicians-who have invested many dollars and years of training in their practices-would be unable to find a suitable alternative profession. The result would be lower payment rates and lower income for physicians. If only a limited number of individuals become physicians due to the large investment required upfront and being faced with the possibility of difficult working conditions and low pay, patients are affected by decreased access to healthcare and longer wait times. Lower payments would mean that physicians would have less money for equipment and less time for patients.

A survey of physicians found that in response to a proposed 10 percent cut in Medicare rates, 28 percent of physicians would stop accepting new Medicare patients, 8 percent would stop treating Medicare patients already under their care, and much higher percentages would discontinue nursing home visits, reduce available hours, or defer investment in medical and health equipment (Book, 2009). This hypothesized response to Medicare and Medicaid restrictions predicts physician response to government-controlled healthcare.

The American Association of Colleges of Nursing (AACN) (2022) reported that the US shortage of nurses is expected to continue to increase as Baby Boomer nurses retire. The Bureau of Labor Statistics projects there will be 175,900 openings for registered nurses through the year 2029. To increase the number of registered nurses, more students need to be accepted into nursing programs. However, a shortage of nursing faculty is restricting nursing program enrollments. According to the AACN (2020), more than 80,000 qualified applicants were rejected in baccalaureate and graduate programs in 2019 due to lack of faculty, clinical sites, classroom space, and clinical preceptors. Two-thirds of respondent schools surveyed indicated shortage of faculty and/or clinical preceptors as reasons for rejecting qualified candidates. Another factor in faculty shortages is the fact that there is higher compensation in clinical and private-sector settings than in higher education (Buerhaus et al., 2017). Nurses who might otherwise be eligible to work as educators are choosing other settings.

The median age for nurses in the US was 52 years in 2021 and the average age of doctorally-prepared faculty is between 51 and 63 years of age (AACN, 2022). Approximately one-third of current nursing faculty in the workforces are expected to retire by 2025 and more than one million nurses are projected to leave the workforce by 2030 (AACN, 2022; Buerhaus et al., 2017). Much of the data on the nursing workforce was collected pre-COVID-19 or early in the pandemic. Even before the pandemic, nursing shortages were identified as factors affecting job satisfaction for nurses and causing many nurses to leave the profession. The pandemic has had a negative effect on nurses entering and staying in the workforce.

Between 2020 and 2022, more nurses reported planning on leaving the workforce than within the past 10 years altogether (Berlin, et al., 2022). A recent survey by Berlin et al. (2022) found that 29 percent of responding RNs in the United States indicated they were likely to leave their current role in direct patient care, with many respondents noting their intent to leave the workforce entirely. Ninety percent of respondents indicated that workforce shortages were a barrier to care (Berlin et al., 2022). US healthcare providers are still experiencing the workforce and operational challenges exacerbated by the pandemic. Patient demand is expected to rise, given the growing and aging population of the United States. Without addressing this potentially wider divide between patient demand and the clinical workforce, with a specific focus on nurses, the US health sector could face substantial repercussions.

If no actions are taken, there will likely be more patients in the United States who will need care than nurses available to deliver it. The US would need to more than double the number of new graduates for the next three years straight to cover the 10 to 20% direct care gap that is projected by 2025. Challenges to meeting this goal are the decreased supply of registered nurses, increasing inpatient demands related to COVID-19 and to a growing and aging population, and changes in work settings.

Government-controlled healthcare delivery systems would exacerbate existing shortages of healthcare providers by decreasing payment rates to hospitals and care providers (Schulman & Milstein, 2014). Limiting the compensation of healthcare professionals may discourage many from entering the health professions (Cannon, 2007). The immediate effect of instituting government-controlled healthcare would be lower incomes for healthcare providers and the reduction of an already declining supply of active healthcare providers, thereby impairing access to healthcare for all patients. This change could affect access and quality of care for future generations (Book, 2009).

Other Workers. Although current shortages of healthcare workers such as doctors and nurses will increase demand and shortages of available providers, many people employed in the private sector of healthcare not working in direct care would see job reductions or elimination of their positions (Araugo & Silberstein, 2022). Government-controlled healthcare could destroy the entire private healthcare sector that represents nearly 20% of our economy (Rosenthal, 2019). Total job losses would be close to 2 million—administrators, coders, billers, claims negotiators, drug and device sales representatives—and have a major impact on the US economy (Rosenthal, 2019). States where healthcare systems employ the largest percentage of the workforce would be more impacted than others (Rosenthal, 2019). Although some job losses would be offset by new positions opened to meet the needs of administration and service in government-controlled healthcare systems, the instability caused by changing systems could affect the US economy for years.

Prices for Services

According to the Kaiser Family Foundation (2012), the actual cost or price of healthcare services in the US may be difficult to determine due to the number of factors involved with pricing. For example, the cost of insurance that can be used to access services consists of premiums, deductions, and out-of-pocket costs (Niles, 2015). These vary depending on the insurance plan and whether it was purchased by an individual, through an employer, or as part of Medicare coverage. Another factor has to do with whether the service is in-network or out-of-network, because insurance companies (and the CMS) negotiate with service providers for payments.

Costs are direct or indirect. Direct costs are the actual cost of delivering the service which also may be difficult to determine because professional fees, staffing, and equipment may be dispersed across direct costs (Partin et al., 2021). A service is considered to be a resource that is used to promote, restore, or maintain health (Partin et al., 2021). Rising costs and a lack of transparency have become two major issues related to healthcare costs today (Banthin, 2018; Blahous, 2018; Finkelman, 2015a).

The solution to reducing costs and increasing transparency is not government-controlled healthcare. Identifying and addressing the root cause of increasing costs so that consumers know the cost of a service before they "purchase" the service would be a start. Restaurants have the prices for food items listed in the menu; grocery stores have prices listed; few consumers would make any major purchase without knowing how much it costs. The same transparency needs to exist for healthcare service costs.

Coverage

Under a federal government-controlled healthcare system, the federal government would have power over the financing and delivery of medical services; it would also determine the benefits and medical procedures that Americans would get, and the prices providers are paid for them (Book, 2009). The absence of competition would give the government-controlled healthcare system the freedom to reduce payments far more than Medicare can in the presence of a large percentage of privately insured patients.

Lower the Quality and Availability of Services

In countries with government-controlled healthcare certain disease treatment outcomes are worse than in the US. The US 5-year survival rate for all cancers is greater than that of Canada, and the United Kingdom (Canadian Cancer Society, 2019; Cancer Research UK, 2018; National Cancer Institute, 2019). The US is ranked first for all OECD countries in discovering and treating cancers in early stages and has higher cancer screening rates for colorectal cancer and cervical cancer that a number of OECD nations (OECD, 2021; Rosenberg, 2018; Thaxter, 2018). All of the comparison countries have government-controlled healthcare.

Government-controlled reimbursements would lead to reduction in quality of care by exacerbating current shortages of physicians, nurses, and other care providers. In the short term, patient access would be limited because current healthcare providers retire earlier or otherwise leave the profession. In the long term, as the prospect of lower lifetime earnings reduces the incentive for people to choose careers in healthcare and there would be fewer healthcare providers to care for an aging population (Book, 2009). Even without the institution of government-controlled healthcare, shortages of healthcare professionals, a growing and aging population, and increased prevalence and incidence of chronic diseases predict dire outcomes for patient care. Changing to government-controlled healthcare would further reduce access and quality of care.

Increased Wait Time for Services. According to the Government Accountability Office (GAO) (2012), more than 9% of Medicaid beneficiaries have had long wait times to get needed care compared to 4% of those with private health insurance. The GAO (2012) reported that part of the wait time or difficulty obtaining care is that more than two-thirds of the states cannot ensure enough Medicaid providers – particularly specialty care providers and dental providers. More than 5% of Medicaid beneficiaries report difficulty obtaining dental services compared to 4% for those who have private insurance. For individuals who are uninsured, more than 12% report difficulty obtaining dental services (GAO, 2012).

There have been inconsistent results in studies examining wait times for services (Araujo & Silberstein, 2022; Aydin et al., 2021; Bengali, 2021; Hussey & Anderson, 2003), however, Canada is an example of a country with national healthcare that has longer wait times for service for both primary care and for specialists than the US (Canadian Institute for Health Information, 2016; Elbaz-Greener et al., 2018; Fox & Poirier, 2018; Merritt Hawkins, 2017). In a comparison of the US, Canada, and several European countries, the Canadian Institute for Health Information (2016) reported that 25% of patients in the US had to wait four weeks to see a specialist compared to 43% in the United Kingdom (UK), 56% in Norway, and 59% in Canada; countries with nationalized healthcare. Almost all countries with government-controlled healthcare have longer wait times for non-emergency care, with Canada having the longest wait times (Wang, 2021). If the US introduced government-controlled healthcare, the shortages of healthcare professionals would reduce access and increase wait times.

Rationing of Healthcare. Healthcare is rationed in many countries with government-controlled healthcare through controlled distribution, budgeting, price setting, and service restrictions (Rattner, 2012; Robinson, 2014; Sussman, 2018). In order to expand coverage countries may use a cost-benefit analysis and the formation of advisory boards to prevent increases in government spending for treatments (Pipes, 2014; *Wall Street Journal*, 2009). According to the *Wall Street Journal* (2009), "once healthcare is nationalized…medical rationing is inevitable."

The fact is that healthcare is already rationed in the US, mainly on the ability to pay. However, rationing in the US is not a top-down centralized policy imposed by the government (Hoffman, 2013). Having a government-controlled healthcare system would mean that government bureaucrats, who are not elected by Americans and often have little to no healthcare background, are making decisions that affect life or death in health-care matters (Hoffman, 2013).

Overuse of Services. When people are provided with government-controlled healthcare and are not directly responsible for the costs of services, they may use more services than needed (Taubman, 2014). The costs to individuals for health insurance needs to be enough to keep people from overusing the system and make setting up appointments for others more difficult (Fisher, 2012). For example, before Medicaid went into effect, people living below the poverty line saw physicians 20% less than those not in poverty (Kelly, 20014). Ten years later, people in poverty receiving Medicaid saw physicians 18% more than those not on Medicaid (Kelly, 2014). In Oregon, 10,000 people who received Medicaid made 40% more visits to emergency rooms, in spite of the fact that they had previously guaranteed access to emergency treatment under federal law (Salsman, 2012; Taubman, 2014).

Values

Americans value independence, self-sufficiency, competition, and being able to make it on their own. Competition between individuals, or between businesses should bring out the best and free enterprise leads to progress (Britannica ProCon, 2019; Cannon, 2007). Americans also believe in action and hard work. People succeed by hard work and work is morally right. The idea of a right to healthcare creates dependence, removes competition and the need to work while providing incentives for using services (Cannon, 2007). The idea of government-controlled healthcare goes against traditional American values.

Attitudes, Beliefs, and Belief Systems

One of the major cons of government-controlled healthcare is that it could lead to socialism. Along with the American values of independence, self-sufficiency, competition, is a foundation of capitalism. Capitalism is an economic and political belief system that favors private ownership of businesses and free markets over government intervention in the economy. Socialism connotes government control of the distribution of goods and services. With a single-payer, centralized healthcare system, everyone has a right to healthcare and healthcare bills are paid by the government. This would give the federal government control over healthcare services. Even in countries like Canada and the UK, the government decides what healthcare treatments individuals are eligible to receive and when they can receive them (Mackey, 2009).

Concern that government involvement in healthcare leads to socialism is not a new argument. In a radio address in 1961, Ronald Reagan spoke out against socialism and socialized medicine. The Kerr-Mills bill that provided "medical care for the aged" had passed in 1960 and there were other proposed bills that would expand the coverage to other populations.

There are many ways in which our government has invaded the precincts of private citizens...this threat is with us, and, at the moment, is...imminent. One of the traditional methods of imposing statism *or socialism on a people has been by way of medicine...under our free enterprise system, we have seen medicine reach the greatest heights that it has in any country in the world. ...This program will pass just as surely as the sun will come up tomorrow; and behind it will come other federal programs that will invade every area of freedom as we have known it in this country. Until, one day...we will awake to find that we have socialism.*

Government-controlled healthcare requires a top-down approach that violates individual freedom and increases the demand for unnecessary services. The free market approach supports individualism and reduces demand for unnecessary services because people will use less of what they have to pay for...Markets are the solution to medical care, just as they are in virtually every other area" (Shapiro, 2017).

Ethics

Ethics provides a systematic, logical framework for analysis, discourse, and decision-making to ensure decisions are grounded. There are several principles that are essential to healthcare ethics. These include respect for persons, beneficence/non maleficence, and justice (National Commission for the Protection of Human Subjects of Biomedical and Behavioral Research, 1979). The principles and examples of ethical dilemmas for healthcare workers are discussed below.

Respect for Persons. The ethical principle, respect for persons, sees every person as having value (Walker, 2015). From the healthcare and research perspective, respect for persons means that everyone should receive information about their health, healthcare, and options for care. The individual should be provided with information in a way that they are able to understand the information and they may then choose whether they want to change behavior, have a surgical procedure, or participate in research.

Respect for persons also includes the concept of autonomy. Autonomy is the right of individuals to self-determination (National Commission for the Protection of Human Subjects of Biomedical and Behavioral Research, 1979). It is the core value of western European and American law and ethics (Walker, 2015). It means that decisions should be made by those affected. The desire of healthcare workers to help others can conflict with autonomy through their desire to take care of people. Additionally, healthcare workers are aware of health behaviors that can lead to health problems and provide education for individuals, families, groups, and communities. Healthcare workers want to help people to be healthier, but they cannot force people to change their behaviors. For example, although the health effects of a fast food diet and inactivity are well-documented, individuals have a personal choice whether to change behaviors (Walker, 2015, p. 80). Education regarding the effects of cigarette smoking on the fetus is important, but as with food and diet, pregnant women have a personal choice of whether to quit smoking.

Government-controlled healthcare would eliminate consumer choice of insurer and other benefits of competition (Blumberg & Holahan, 2019). If all Americans are on the same government-controlled healthcare plan and private insurers are not allowed, there is no choice. In addition, in trying to meet the needs of "all Americans," some populations would not have their needs met because everyone's healthcare needs are not the same, it will take away the right of individuals to self-determination. Individuals will be told which care providers they can see whether or not they can have elective procedures and which medications they can take. In these ways, government-controlled healthcare can violate autonomy. Will scarcity of healthcare workers, cost containment and reductions lead to rationing of care based on whether or not patients are compliant with "good" health behaviors?

Beneficence/Nonmaleficence. Beneficence is the desire to act in the best interest of others and is the strongest guiding principle of healthcare professionals (National Commission for the Protection of Human Subjects of Biomedical and Behavioral Research, 1979). A conflict or dilemma occurs when the desire to help (beneficence) conflicts with respect for the other person's right to choose for themselves (autonomy). One example of a government-controlled healthcare program is CHIP. CHIP was developed to provide care for children . The supporters of CHIP saw the program as beneficial for children's health. When data indicated a decrease in participation in the Children's Health Insurance Program (CHIP), no one could understand why parents would refuse the benefits of a program such as CHIP. However, research found that the $50 enrollment fee was a barrier because parents could not see spending the money if their child was not sick and if their child became sick, they could go to the emergency room for treatment for free.

Nonmaleficence is the other side of beneficence. While beneficence is concerned with doing good; nonmaleficence is concerned with not doing harm (National Commission for the Protection of Human Subjects of Biomedical and Behavioral Research, 1979). It is important to evaluate what harm might result from interventions. What responses might parents have to government-controlled healthcare? If government-controlled healthcare is delivered like CHIP, parents may not perceive it beneficial to participate. If the government controls healthcare, will decisions made by the government harm the relationship between the parent and child? Parents have become more concerned about the role of government in their children's lives. The current concern is that children are being taught ideas in public schools that are not consistent with the values and beliefs of parents. Would government-controlled healthcare be any less of a concern than government-controlled education?

Justice. Justice is the fair distribution of rights and resources. Allocation is considered by what is fair and of greatest benefit to the most people. The concepts of justice are commonly understood as (1) to each person an equal share, (2) to each person according to individual need, (3) to each person according to individual effort, (4) to each person according to societal contribution, and (5) to each person according to merit (National Commission for the Protection of Human Subjects of Biomedical and Behavioral Research, 1979). Justice also incorporates how decisions are made regarding the allocation of scarce goods and services. When there are reductions in human services programs due to budget cuts, choices may be made based on the perceived worth of the individuals/communities. As the cost of healthcare increases, so does the population of uninsured and underinsured. Again, the question of who will make decisions and how they will be made regarding care is one of justice. Trends like this have increased the movement to force participation in some form of health insurance or other payment plan. As resources become more scarce and demand increases, this and other restrictive trends would likely be suggested.

CONCLUSION

While most Americans have access to some level of health insurance, they do not have a choice of health plans that provide personalized, patient-centered care, meaning the kind of health coverage and care that they personally choose and control and that is directly accountable to them. Key decisions on the kinds of health plans, benefits, and payment arrangements that are available are legally reserved to government officials, corporate human resources officials, or health insurance executives.

The US is in dire need of changes in the healthcare system. This is not questioned by either the pro government-controlled healthcare side or the con government-controlled healthcare side. The question is whether incremental changes can be made to the current system that are acceptable to everyone or whether the current system should be thrown out and replaced with government-controlled healthcare. A total government takeover of the healthcare system would be a monumental and disruptive enterprise. It would be an unprecedented expansion of government power, and it would inevitably increase costs and the burdens on providers, stifle innovation, and limit access to high-quality care, especially for patients in need of complex and technologically advanced medical services (Moffitt, n. d.).

For all Americans, at issue is whether their healthcare is to be government-controlled and centralized, or whether healthcare financing and delivery is to be driven by the decisions of individuals in consultation with their doctors in a free market governed by consumer choice and competition. Who decides?

REFERENCES

Altenstetter, C. (2003). Insights from healthcare in Germany. *American Journal of Public Health, 93*(1), 38–44. doi:10.2105/AJPH.93.1.38 PMID:12511381

American Association of Colleges of Nursing (2020). 2019-2020 enrollment and graduations in baccalaureate and graduate programs in nursing.

American Association of Colleges of Nursing. (2022). *Fact sheet: Nursing shortage.* https://www.aacnnursing.org/news-information/fact-sheets/nursing-shortage

Anderson, E. T. (2015). Community health nursing: Essentials of practice. In E. T. Anderson & J. McFarlane (Eds.), *Community as partner: Theory and practice in nursing* (7th ed., pp. 19–28). Wolters Kluwer.

Araujo, M., & Silberstein, S. (2022). What is single-payer health insurance? *The Balance/Dotdash Meredith.* https://www.thebalance.com/is-single-payer-health-insurance-a-good-deal-how-does-anthinit-work-4175823

Aydin, S., Collins, S. K., Puja, J. H. A., & Nash, J. K. (2021). Evaluation of US and Taiwan health system performance: A review of the literature. *International Journal of Health Management and Tourism, 6*(1), 415–426. https://dergipark.org.tr/tr/pub/ijhmt. doi:10.31201/ijhmt.834649

Banthin, J. (2018, May 24). *Projections of federal spending on major healthcare programs* [Paper presentation]. Alliance for Health Policy Summit on Healthcare Costs in America. Washington, DC, United States.

Barua, B., Jacques, D., & Collyer, A. (2018). Waiting your turn: Wait times for healthcare in Canada, 2018 report. *Fraser Institute.* https://www.fraserinstitute.org/studies/waiting-your-turn-wait-times-for-health-care-in-canada-2018

Bengali, S. M. (2021). *A comparison of hospital capacities between single-payer and multi-payer healthcare systems among OECD nations* (Publication No. 28418466) [Master's thesis, Purdue University]. Georgetown ProQuest Dissertations Publishing.

Berlin, G., Lapointe, M., Murphy, M., & Wexler, J. (2022, May 11). Assessing the lingering impact of COVID-19 on the nursing workforce. McKinsey & Company. https://www.mckinsey.com/industries/healthcare-systems-and-services/our-insights/assessing-the-lingering-impact-of-covid-19-on-the-nursing-workforce

Blahous, C. (2018, July 30). The costs of a national single-payer healthcare system. Mercatus Research Paper. https://ssrn.com/abstract=3232864. doi:10.2139/ssrn.3232864

Blumberg, L. J., & Holahan, J. (2019). *The pros and cons of single-payer health plans*. Urban Institute.

Book, R. (2009). Single payer: Why government-run-health-care will harm both patients and doctors. *The Heritage Foundation.* https://www.heritage.org/health-care-reform/report/single-payer-why-government-run-health-care-will-harm-both-patients-and-doctors

Buerhaus, P. I., Auerbach, D. I., & Staiger, D. O. (2017, May 3). How should we prepare for the wave of retiring Baby Boomer nurses? *Health Affairs.* https://www.healthaffairs.org/do/10.1377/forefront.20170503.059894/full/

Canadian Cancer Society. (2019). *Cancer statistics at a glance*. Canadian Cancer Society. https://cancer.ca/en/research/cancer-statistics/cancer-statistics-at-a-glance

Canadian Institute for Health Information. (2016). How Canada compares: Results from the commonwealth fund's 2016 international health policy survey of adults in 11 countries. *The Commonwealth Fund.* https://www.commonwealthfund.org/publications

Cancer Research UK. (2019). *Cancer survival statistics for all cancers combined.* https://www.cancerresearchuk.org/health-professional/cancer-statistics/survival

Cannon, M. F. (2007, June 29). A 'right' to healthcare? *National Review Online.* https://www.nationalreview.com/2007/06/right-health-care-michael-f-cannon/

Chansatitporn, N., & Pobkeeree, V. (2020). Leadership and quality management measurement models: An empirical study. *International Journal of Health Care Quality Assurance, 33*(1), 52–66. doi:10.1108/IJHCQA-07-2019-0118 PMID:31898882

Chernew, M., & Mintz, H. (2021). Administrative expenses in the US healthcare system: Why so high? *Journal of the American Medical Association, 326*(17), 1679–1680. doi:10.1001/jama.2021.17318 PMID:34668530

Committee for a Responsible Federal Budget. (2016, May 19). *Adding up Senator Sanders's campaign proposals far.* https://www.crfb.org/papers/adding-senator-sanderss-campaign-proposals-so-far

Committee on the Robert Wood Johnson Foundation Initiative on the Future of Nursing. (2011). The future of nursing: Leading change, advancing health. National Academies Press (US). doi:10.17226/12956

Curtis, P., Vizzini, D., & Church, B. (2022). *The Colorado multi-payer collaborative: A framework for integration of whole-person care*. Milbank Memorial Fund.

Dao, A., & Mulligan, J. (2016). Toward an anthropology of insurance and health reform. *Medical Anthropology Quarterly*, *30*(1), 5–17. doi:10.1111/maq.12271 PMID:26698645

De Lew, N., Greenberg, G., & Kinchen, K. (1992). A layman's guide to the U.S. healthcare system. *Health Care Financing Review*, *4*(1), 51–69.

Diamond, M. A. (2009). Con: Single-payer healthcare: Why it's not the best answer. *American Journal of Respiratory and Critical Care Medicine*, *180*, 921–922. doi:10.1164/rccm.200906-0882ED PMID:19897772

Draper, D. A., Fellandy, L. E., Liebhaber, A., & Lauer, J. R. (2008). Massachusetts reform: High costs and expanding expectations may weaken employer support. *Issue Brief (Center for Studying Health System Change)*, *124*, 1–6. PMID:19024889

Elbaz-Greener, G., Yarranton, B., Qiu, F., Wood, D. A., Webb, J. G., Fremes, S. E., Radhakrishnan, S., & Wijeysundera, H. C. (2019). Association between wait time for transcatheter aortic valve replacement and early postprocedural outcomes. *Journal of the American Heart Association*, *8*(1), e010407. doi:10.1161/JAHA.118.010407 PMID:30612506

Field, C. (2011, March 4). Ronald Reagan fought against Obamacare 50 years before it became law. *Townhall.* https://townhall.com/tipsheet/chrisfield/2011/03/04/ronald-reagan-fought-against-obamacare-50-years-before-it-became-law-n683529

Finkelman, A. W. (2015a). Economics of healthcare. In M. A. Nies & M. McEwen (Eds.), *Community/public health nursing: Promoting the health of populations* (6th ed., pp. 202–219). Elsevier.

Finkelman, A. W. (2015b). The healthcare system. In M. A. Nies & M. McEwen (Eds.), *Community/public health nursing: Promoting the health of populations* (6th ed., pp. 186–201). Elsevier.

Fisher, S. (April 6, 2022). Medicare for all: Definition and pros and cons. *SmartAsset.* https://smartasset.com/insurance/medicare-for-all-definition-and-pros-and-cons

Fox, A., & Poirier, R. (2018). How single-payer stacks up: Evaluating different models of universal health coverage on cost, access, and quality. *International Journal of Health Services, 48*(3), 568–585. doi:10.1177/0020731418779377 PMID:29925286

Francis, P. (2016, May 9). Healthcare is a 'universal right,' not a 'consumer good.' *Catholic Culture.* https://www.catholicculture.org/news/headlines/index.cfm?storyid=28266&repos=4&subrepos=2&searchid=2231158

Friedman, G. (2021). *Funding universal healthcare in the Commonwealth of Massachusetts: Replacing an inefficient, inequitable, and destructive healthcare finance system with a fair system that will promote economic efficiency and better health* [Unpublished manuscript]. Department of Economics, University of Massachusetts at Amherst.

Galvani, A. P., Parpia, A. S., Foster, E. M., Singer, B. H., & Fitzpatrick, M. C. (2020) Improving the prognosis of healthcare in the USA. *Lancet, 15*(395)(10223), 524-533. . PMID: 32061298; PMCID: PMC8572548. doi:10.1016/S0140-6736(19)33019-3

Gregory, P. R. (2013, October 28). Obamacare a mess? Liberals say go single payer. *Forbes.* https://www.forbes.com/sites/paulroderickgregory/2013/10/28/obama-care-a-mess-liberals-say-go-single-payer/?sh=3e5746ac28a0

Gudbranson, E., Glickman, A., & Emanuel, E. J. (2017). Reassessing the data on whether a physician shortage exists. *Journal of the American Medical Association, 317*(19), 1945–1946. doi:10.1001/jama.2017.2609 PMID:28319245

Heath, S. (2017). *Physician shortage drives wait times, harms patient care access.* Xtelligent Healthcare Media. https://patientengagementhit.com/news/physician-shortage-drives-wait-times-harms-patient-care-access

Henderson Gist, J. (2015). Partnering with communities for healthy public policy. In E. T. Anderson & J. McFarlane (Eds.), *Community as partner: Theory and practice in nursing* (7th ed., pp. 116–126). Wolters Kluwer.

Higgins Donius, M. A. (2011). Public health: Costs, challenges, and considerations. In M. Truglio-Londrigan & S. B. Lewenson (Eds.), *Public health nursing: Practicing population-based care* (pp. 347–358). Jones and Bartlett.

Hoffman, B. (2013, January 18). Healthcare rationing is nothing new. *Scientific American.* https://www.scientificamerican.com/article/health-care-rationing-is/

Holahan, J., Buettgens, M., Clemons-Cope, L., Favreault, M. M., Blumberg, L. J., & Ndwandwe, S. (2016). *The Sanders single-payer healthcare plan: Effect on national health expenditures and federal private spending*. Urban Institute.

Huguet, N., Angier, H., Hoopes, M. J., Marino, M., Heintzman, J., Schmidt, T., & DeVoe, J. E. (2019). Prevalence of pre-existing conditions among community health center patients before and after the affordable care act. *Journal of the American Board of Family Medicine*, *32*(6), 883–889. doi:10.3122/jabfm.2019.06.190087 PMID:31704757

Hussey, P., & Anderson, G. F. (2003). A comparison of single-and-multi-payer health insurance systems and options for reform. *Health Policy (Amsterdam)*, *66*(3), 215–228. doi:10.1016/S0168-8510(03)00050-2 PMID:14637007

Kaiser Family Foundation. (2012). *The uninsured: A primer.* https://kff.org/uninsured/report/the-uninsured-a-primer-key-facts-about-health-insurance-on-the-eve-of-coverage-expansions

Kambil, A. (2017, January 5). Managing the execution risks of change initiatives. *The Wall Street Journal.* https://deloitte.wsj.com/articles/managing-the-execution-risks-of-change-initiatives-1483678935

Kelly, D. (2010, May 12). Is there a right to healthcare? *Atlas Society.* https://www.atlassociety.org/post/is-there-a-right-to-health-care

Korobkin, R. (2014). Comparative effectiveness research as choice architecture: The behavioral law and economics solution to the healthcare cost crisis. *Michigan Law Review*. https://repository.law.umich.edu/mlr/vol112/iss4/1

Kwapisz, A. (2020). Health insurance coverage and sources of advice in entrepreneurship: Gender differences. *Journal of Business Venturing Insights*, *14*, e00177. doi:10.1016/j.jbvi.2020.e00177

Lapidus, J. (2017). Private health insurance in Sweden: Fast-track lanes and the alleged attempts to stop them. *Health Policy (Amsterdam)*, *121*(4), 442–449. doi:10.1016/j.healthpol.2017.02.004 PMID:28228243

Long, S. K. (2008). On the road to universal coverage: Impacts of reforming Massachusetts at one year. *Health Affairs (Project Hope)*, *27*(Suppl1), w270–w284. doi:10.1377/hlthaff.27.4.w270 PMID:18522948

Mackey, J. (2009). The Whole Foods Alternative to ObamaCare. *Wall Street Journal, 11*.

Masterson, L. (2017). CBO reports show private insurers pay physicians, hospitals far more than Medicare. *Healthcare Dive*. https://www.healthcaredive.com/news/cbo-reports-show-private-insurers-pay-physicians-hospitals-far-more-than-m/445949/

McArdle, M. (2016, August 23). Healthcare is a business, not a right. *Bloomberg View*. https://www.bloomberg.com/opinion/articles/2016-08-23/health-care-is-a-business-not-a-right

McGrath, N., Foley, B., Hurley, C., Ryan, M., & Flynn, R. (2022). A multi-method quality improvement approach to systematically improve and promote the quality of national health and social care information. *The HIM Journal*, *51*(1), 50–56. doi:10.1177/1833358320926422 PMID:32586137

Merritt Hawkins Team. (2017). 2017 survey of physician appointment wait times and Medicare and Medicaid acceptance rates. *Merritt Hawkins*. https://www.merritthawkins.com/news-and-insights/thought-leadership/survey/survey-of-physician-appointment-wait-times/

Moffitt, R. (n. d.). The truth about government-controlled healthcare. *The Heritage Foundation*. https://www.heritage.org/article/the-truth-about-government-controlled-health-care

Montgomery, K. (2022). Single-payer healthcare vs. universal coverage. *Verywellhealth*. https://www/verywellhealth.com/difference-between-universal-coverage-and-single-payer-system-1738546

Myer, C. R. (2007). Failed promises: The demise of the original TennCare vision. *Managed Care Interface*, *20*, 24–30. PMID:17405578

National Cancer Institute. (2019). Cancer stat facts: Cancer of any site. *Seer*. https://seer.cancer.gov/statfacts/html/all.html

National Commission for the Protection of Human Subjects of Biomedical and Behavioral Research. (1979). *The Belmont report: Ethical principles and guidelines for the protection of human subjects of research*. U.S. Department of Health and Human Services. https://www.hhs.gov/ohrp/regulations-and-policy/belmont-report/read-the-belmont-report/index.html

Niles, N. (2015). *Basics of the U. S. healthcare system* (2nd ed.). Jones and Bartlett.

Nunn, R., Parsons, J., & Shambaugh, J. (2020). A dozen facts about the economics of the U. S. health-care system. *The Hamilton Project: Brookings*. https://www.brookings.edu/research/a-dozen-facts-about-the-economics-of-the-u-s-health-care-system/

Organization for Economic Cooperation and Development (OECD) (2021). *Health at a Glance: 2021 indicators.* oecd.org

Parascandola, M. (1996). Evidence and association: Epistemic confusion in toxic tort law. *Philosophy of Science, 63*(S3), S168–S176. doi:10.1086/289949

Parker, J. D., Talih, M., Malec, D. J., Beresovsky, V. B., Carroll, M., Gonzalez, J. F., Jr., Hamilton, B. E., Ingram, D. D., Kochanek, K., McCarty, F., Moriarity, C., Shimizu, I., Strashny, A., & Ward, B. W. (2017). *National center for health statistics data presentation standards for proportions.* National Center for Health Statistics. https://www.cdc.gov/nchs/data/series/sr_02/sr02_175.pdf

Paul, R. (2010, July 19). Healthcare is not a right. *Russia Today (RT).* rt.com

ProCon.org (2019). Should all Americans have the right (be entitled) to healthcare? *Britannica ProCon.* http://healthcare.procon.org

Rattner, S. (2012, September 16). Beyond Obamacare. *New York Times.* https://www.nytimes.com/2012/09/17/opinion/health-care-reform-beyond-obamacare.html

Reagan, R. (1961). Socialized Medicine [Radio address transcribed audio recording]. *American Rhetoric.* https://www.americanrhetoric.com/speeches/ronaldreagansocializedmedicine.htm

Robinson, S. (2014, January 31). GPs warn of rise of rationing. *GPOnline.* https://www.gponline.com/exclusive-gps-warn-rise-rationing/article/1229380

Rosenberg, J. (2018, July 31). Cancer screening rates in the US fall short of Healthy People 2020 targets. *AJMC.* https://www.ajmc.com/view/cancer-screening-rates-in-the-us-fall-short-of-healthy-people-2020-targets

Rosenthal, E. (2019, May 24). Analysis: A healthcare overhaul could kill 2 million jobs, and that's ok. *Kaiser Health News.* https://khn.org/news/analysis-a-health-care-overhaul-could-kill-2-million-jobs-and-thats-ok/

Roy, A. (2013, August 10). Senator Harry Reid: Obamacare 'absolutely' a step toward a single-payer system. https://www.forbes.com/sites/theapothecary/2013/08/10/sen-harry-reid-obamacare-absolutely-a-step-toward-a-single-payer-system/?sh=5e91c5973af9

Ryan, P. (2011). Healthcare reform: The way forward. *Notre Dame Journal of Law, Ethics & Public Policy, 25*(2), 337–353. https://scholarship.law.nd.edu/ndjlepp/vol25/iss2/3

Salsman, R. M, (2012, April 3). Memo to the Supreme Court: Healthcare is not a right. *Forbes.*

Sanders, B. (2017, February 10). Issues: Healthcare as a human right--Medicare for all. https://berniesanders.com/issues/medicare-for-all/

Scheinker, D., Richman, B. D., Milstein, A., & Schulman, K. A. (2021). Reducing administrative costs in US healthcare: Assessing single payer and its alternatives. *Health Services Research, 56*(4), 615–625. doi:10.1111/1475-6773.13649 PMID:33788283

Schulman, K. A., & Milstein, A. (2019). The implications of "Medicare for All" for US hospitals. *Journal of the American Medical Association, 321*(17), 1661. doi:10.1001/jama.2019.3134 PMID:30946429

Shapiro, B. (2017). Healthcare is a commodity, not a right. *National Review*, 11.

Shultz, C. M., & Kelley, K. (2011). Nursing education and public health nursing. In M. Truglio-Londrigan & S. B. Lewenson (Eds.), *Public health nursing: Practicing population-based care* (pp. 359–384). Jones and Bartlett.

Statista Research Department. (2022). Health insurance in the United States—Statistics and facts. Statista. *Statista.* https://www.statista.com/topics/7807/health-insurance-in-the-us/#dossierKeyfigures

Straube, B. M. (2012). A role for government: An observation on federal healthcare efforts in prevention. *American Journal of Preventive Medicine, 44*(1S1), S39-S42. doi:10.1016/j.amepre.2012.09.009

Sussman, M. (2018, March 6). Do fixed cost-effectiveness thresholds or CE threshold magnitude matter? *Panalgo.* https://blog.panalgo.com/blog/fixed-cost-effectiveness-thresholds

Taubman, S. L., Allen, H. L., Wright, B. J., Baicker, K., & Finkelstein, A. N. (2014). Medicaid increases emergency department use: Evidence from Oregon's health insurance experiment. *Science, 343*(6168), 263–268. doi:10.1126cience.1246183 PMID:24385603

Thaxter, M. (2018). UK cancer survival rates still trailing European peers. *Deloitte.* https://blogs.deloitte.co.uk/health/2018/02/uk-cancer-survival-rates-still-trailing-european-peers.html

Thorpe, K. E. (2016). An analysis of Senator Sanders's single payer plan [Unpublished manuscript]. Finance, Emory University.

Turati, G. (2013). The Italian Servizio Sanitario Nazionale: A renewing tale of lost promises. In J. Costa-Font, & S. L. Greer, S.L. (Eds.) Federalism and decentralization in European health and social care (pp. 47-66). Palgrave Macmillan. doi:10.1057/9781137291875_3

United States Bureau of Labor Statistics. (2022). *Occupational outlook handbook: Registered Nurses*. USBLS. https://www.bls.gov/ooh/healthcare/registered-nurses.htm

United States Government Accountability Office. (2012, November). *Medicaid: States made multiple program changes, and beneficiaries generally reported access comparable to private insurance* (GAO-13-55). https://www.gao.gov/products/gao-13-55

Walker, S. S. (2015). Ethical quandaries in community health nursing. In E. T. Anderson & J. McFarlane (Eds.), *Community as partner: Theory and practice in nursing* (7th ed., pp. 74–86). Wolters Kluwer.

Wall Street Journal. (2009, November 1). The worst bill ever: Epic new spending and taxes, pricier insurance, rationed care, dishonest accounting: The Pelosi health bill has it all. *Wall Street Journal*. https://www.wsj.com/articles/SB10001424052748703399204574505423751140690

Wang, E. (2021). Universal healthcare: An argument for a US transition in light of COVID-19. *Journal of Interdisciplinary Public Policy*, *2*(2), 3–11.

WHO. (2013). *The world health report 2013: Research for universal health coverage*. WHO. https://www.who.int/publications/i/item/9789240690837

World Health Organization (WHO). (1978). *Declaration of Alma-Ata, 1978*. WHO. http://www.who.int/hpr/ NPH/docs/declaration_almaata.pdf

Zhang, X., Tai, D., Pforsich, H., & Lin, V. W. (2018). United States registered nurse workforce report card and shortage forecast: A revisit. *The American Journal of Medicine*, *33*(3), 229–236. doi:10.1177/1062860617738328 PMID:29183169

Chapter 3
Towards a Comprehensive National Health System for the United States

David Stewart
Winston-Salem State University, USA

Sheilia R. Goodwin
Winston-Salem State University, USA

Nikolaos Karagiannis
Winston-Salem State University, USA

ABSTRACT

This chapter first provides the two main theoretical perspectives related to the U.S. health system: the "market-based" view and the "socially sensitive" argument. The second main section discusses important facts and highlights related to the national health situation of the United States compared with other advanced OECD countries. Taking these facts and highlights into consideration, the final sections of the contribution critically examine the merits and demerits of contrasting approaches to implementing a comprehensive national health and insurance scheme in the United States, and offer concrete policy considerations. Some brief conclusions end the chapter.

DOI: 10.4018/978-1-6684-4060-5.ch003

INTRODUCTION

Healthcare in the United States is provided through a combination of private health insurance and public health coverage (e.g., Medicare, Medicaid). Based on latest statistics, around 45 percent of health spending is paid for by the government at either the federal or state and local level. According to the Centers for Medicare & Medicaid Services (CMS Program Statistics, 2018), in 2017, the U.S. health spending reached $3,492.1 billion or approximately $10,740 *per capita*, and accounted for 17.9 percent of the nation's Gross Domestic Product (see Figure 1: CMS, 2018). U.S. hospitals are largely owned and operated by private sector institutions with 3.3 percent being federal and 15.7 percent being state and local government or community hospitals (Figure 2: American Hospital Association, 2019). Further, 47.8 percent are nongovernment not-for-profit, 21.3 percent are for-profit, and 11.9 percent are non-federal psychiatric and "other" hospitals. Although nearly 45 percent of healthcare spending and close to 18 percent of acute care facilities are government-supported (CMS, 2018), the U.S. does not have a universal healthcare system. This contributes to health disparities when the U.S. is compared to other advanced industrial countries (OECD, 2018).

Moreover, the United States life expectancy is 78.6 years at birth, up from 75.2 years in 1990; this ranks 22nd out of the 35 industrialized OECD countries, down from 20th in 1990 (OECD, 2018, 2020). A relatively recent CDC statement (Nov 15, 2019), however, indicates U.S. life expectancy has been reduced by drug overdoses and suicides over the past several years. Of 17 high-income countries studied by the National Institutes of Health, in 2018, the United States had the highest or near-highest prevalence of obesity, car accidents, infant mortality, heart and lung disease, sexually transmitted infections, adolescent pregnancies, homicides, and injuries (NIH, 2019). A 2018 survey of the healthcare systems of 11 developed countries found that the U.S. healthcare system to be the most expensive and worst-performing in terms of health access, efficiency, and equity (OECD, Health Statistics 2019). While real incomes remained almost stagnant during the last two decades, health expenses have increased enormously.

What's more, in 2018, there were nearly 41 million people and around 28 million families living in poverty in the United States with blacks and Hispanics experiencing the highest poverty rates. Prohibitively high cost is the primary reason Americans have problems accessing healthcare . Based on statistics by the U.S. Census Bureau and the Gallup organization, around 29 million did not have health insurance in 2018 (U.S. Census Bureau, Annual Social and Economic Supplements, 2018, 2019). Such a large number of people without health insurance coverage in the United States is one of the primary concerns raised by advocates of healthcare reform.

With such a general background in mind, the article, first, provides the two main theoretical perspectives related to the U.S. health system: the "market-based" view and the "socially sensitive" argument. The second section discusses important facts and highlights related to the national health situation of the United States. Taking these facts and highlights into consideration, the final sections of the article critically examine the merits and demerits of contrasting approaches to implementing a national health and insurance scheme in the U.S., and offer concrete policy considerations. Some brief conclusions end the article.

THEORETICAL PERSPECTIVES

In the United States, there have been two broad sets of argument related to adopting "a national health and insurance scheme" ("Medicare-for-All" or "universal single-payer system"), particularly during the last decade: the first, the "market-based" argument, relies heavily on the neoclassical marginal analysis and the "dollars-and-cents" logic; and the second, the "socially-sensitive" approach, emphasizes important principles such as coverage of the health needs of the total population and "social justice".

According to the proponents of the "market-based" view, mandatory health insurance increases the role of government as well as the expenses associated with a comprehensive national health and insurance scheme, provides perverse incentives for employers, is heavily subsidized, restrains individual choices, utilizes the "carrot and stick" approach, and offers limited results (e.g., uninsured individuals typically receive less care in a given year and wait longer to get treated). Mandatory healthcare can result in fewer uninsured but cannot contain fast rising costs in the healthcare system. Growing burdens on businesses mean that an increasing number may choose to steer employees into the mandatory health system rather than provide health insurance themselves. Consequently, market incentives are crucial to solve the pressing problems of efficiency and cost containment (Richardson, 2011). Some experts also point out countries, such as Singapore and the Netherlands, that have introduced "managed competition" in health services provision.

There are additional important issues associated with this view. One key issue is the social and political culture in America. Survey research conducted by the International Social Survey Program has found that a lower percentage of Americans believe that healthcare for the sick is a government responsibility than citizens in other advanced countries like Canada, the U.K., Germany or Sweden (ISSP, 2011). Another important reason is the role of interest groups in influencing the political process. A third reason the U.S. lacks universal health coverage is that America's political institutions make it difficult for massive entitlement programs to be enacted.

As policy experts have pointed out in studies of the U.S. health system, the country does not have a comprehensive national health insurance system because "American political institutions are structurally biased against this kind of comprehensive reform" (Schuck & Wilson, 2008, p. x). The political system is prone to inertia and any attempt at comprehensive reform must pass through the obstacles of congressional committees, budget estimates, conference committees, amendments, and a potential veto while opponents of reform may publicly condemn the bill (Bond & Smith, 2016). Lobbyism is playing a substantial role in the inertia as well.

Ultimately, the U.S. remains the only advanced industrialized nation without a comprehensive national health insurance system because of the many ways America is exceptional. The U.S. culture is remarkably individualistic favoring personal initiatives over government responsibility; lobbyists are particularly active spending billions to ensure that private insurers maintain their status in the health system; and institutions are designed in a manner that limits major welfare programs and social policy changes (Bond & Smith, 2016).

According to the "socially-sensitive" line of argument, a number of studies confirm that prices and administrative costs in the U.S. are significantly higher compared with developed countries that have some type of single-payer system. In a 2003 study, Anderson, Hussey and Petrosyan argued that prices account for much of the higher healthcare spending in the U.S. This is particularly disturbing when considering that real wages have remained almost stagnant during the last 20 years or so while healthcare prices have gone up excessively and disproportionately. A more recent study (Anderson, Hussey, & Petrosyan, 2019) confirmed the results of their earlier study, despite all the reforms that have occurred since 2003, including Obamacare. Papanicolas, Woskie and Jha (2018) reached a similar conclusion that, "the United States spent approximately twice as much as other high-income countries on medical care". Nor do Americans receive more care –in fact, by some measures they actually receive less care (fewer visits to physicians, for example). However, the country is still spending more; a difference that is largely explained by higher prices. The 2019 study by Anderson et al. further demonstrated that the difference between prices paid in the private and public sectors has widened considerably since 2003. It is the greater dependence on private payers, rather than on government as single payer, that accounts for higher costs. Despite the increasing costs of healthcare in the U.S., the country is among the poorest performers in providing healthcare among industrialized nations.

Prohibitively high cost is the primary reason Americans have problems accessing healthcare . The rate of adults uninsured for healthcare peaked at 18.0 percent in 2013 prior to the ACA mandate, fell to 10.9 percent in the third quarter of 2016, and stood at 13.7 percent in the fourth quarter of 2018, based on surveys by the Gallup organization beginning in 2008 (Gallup Personal Health Issues, 2020). At over 40 million, the number of people without health insurance coverage in the United States is one of the primary concerns raised by advocates of healthcare reform. Lack of health insurance is associated with increased mortality, about sixty thousand preventable deaths per year, depending on the study reviewed. Studies done at Harvard Medical School indicated that millions of Americans skip medications due to their high cost, and nearly 45,000 annual deaths are associated with a lack of patient health insurance. Studies also found that uninsured, working Americans have an approximately 40 percent higher mortality risk compared to privately insured working Americans (Harvard Health Publishing, various).

Administrative costs in the United States also contribute to rising healthcare costs. For instance, governance and administration costs accounted for 8 percent of total national health expenditures in the U.S. compared to a range of 1 to 3 percent in the other countries (Papanicolas, Woskie, & Jha (2018) calculated an OECD average of about 3 percent). What is more, administrative costs on the provider side are estimated to be high in the U.S. as well. For instance, over 24 percent of U.S. hospital spending is on administration, compared to around 13 percent in Canada.

IMPORTANT FACTS: HIGHLIGHTS

The U.S. healthcare system is notorious for its high costs and below par outcomes. The highlights in the following paragraphs are based on historical and projected national expenditures collected in the last five years as well as on international comparisons between the U.S. and other advanced OECD countries between 1970 and 2018 (CDC, 2018; CMS, 2018, 2019; U.S. Census Bureau, 2018, 2019).

Historical NHE, 2019

- In 2017, 8.8 percent of the U.S. population, or 28.5 million people, did not have health insurance at any point during the year as measured by the Current Population Survey–Annual Social and Economic Supplement. The uninsured rate and number of uninsured people in 2017 were not statistically different from 2016 (8.8 percent or 28.1 million).
- The percentage of people with health insurance coverage for all or part of 2017 was 91.2 percent, not statistically different from the rate in 2016. Between 2016 and 2017, the number of people with health insurance coverage increased by 2.3 million, up to 294.6 million.
- In 2017, private health insurance coverage continued to be more prevalent than government coverage, at 67.2 percent and 37.7 percent, respectively. Of the sub-types of health insurance coverage, employer-based insurance was

the most common, covering 56.0 percent of the population for some or all the calendar year, followed by Medicaid (19.3 percent), Medicare (17.2 percent), direct-purchase coverage (16.0 percent), and military coverage (4.8 percent).

- Between 2016 and 2017, the rate of Medicare coverage increased by 0.6 percentage points to cover 17.2 percent of people for part or all of 2017 (up from 16.7 percent in 2016). However, managed care, where payers use various techniques intended to improve quality and limit cost, has become ubiquitous.
- The military coverage rate increased by 0.2 percentage points to 4.8 percent during this time. Coverage rates for employment-based coverage, direct-purchase coverage, and Medicaid did not statistically change between 2016 and 2017.
- In 2017, the percentage of uninsured children under age 19 (5.4 percent) was not statistically different from the percentage in 2016. For children under age 19 in poverty, the uninsured rate (7.8 percent) was higher than for children not in poverty (4.9 percent).
- Across different States, disparities in healthcare and health outcomes are widespread. Minorities are more likely to suffer from serious illnesses and less likely to have access to quality healthcare, including preventative services. Between 2016 and 2017, the percentage of people without health insurance coverage at the time of interview decreased in three states and increased in 14 states. Between 2016 and 2017, the uninsured rate did not statistically change for any race or Hispanic origin group. In 2017, non-Hispanic Whites had the lowest uninsured rate among race and Hispanic-origin groups (6.3 percent). The uninsured rates for Blacks and Asians were 10.6 percent and 7.3 percent, respectively. Hispanics had the highest uninsured rate (16.1 percent).
- The U.S. life expectancy is 78.6 years at birth, up from 75.2 years in 1990; this ranks 42nd among 224 nations, and 22nd out of the 35 industrialized OECD countries, down from 20th in 1990. In 2016 and 2017, life expectancy in the U.S. dropped for the first time since 1993. Of 17 high-income countries studied by the National Institutes of Health, in 2017, the United States had the highest or near-highest prevalence of obesity, car accidents, infant mortality, heart and lung disease, sexually transmitted infections, adolescent pregnancies, injuries, and homicides. Still, the underutilization of preventative measures, rates of preventable illness, and prevalence of chronic disease suggest that the U.S. healthcare system does not sufficiently promote wellness (CMS, National Health Expenditure Data: Historical, 2019).

Projected NHE, 2018-2027

- Under current law, national health spending is projected to grow at an average rate of 5.5 percent per year for 2018-27 and to reach nearly $6.0 trillion by 2027.
- Health spending is projected to grow 0.8 percentage point faster than Gross Domestic Product (GDP) per year over the 2018-27 period; as a result, the health share of GDP is expected to rise from 17.9 percent in 2017 to 19.4 percent by 2027.
- Key economic and demographic factors fundamental to the health sector are anticipated to be the major drivers during 2018-27.
- Prices for healthcare goods and services are projected to grow somewhat faster over 2018-27 (2.5 percent compared to 1.1 percent for 2014-17).
- As a result of comparatively higher projected enrollment growth, average annual spending growth in Medicare (7.4 percent) is expected to exceed that of Medicaid (5.5 percent) and private health insurance (4.8 percent).
- The Medicare enrollment impacts are the key reason the share of healthcare spending sponsored by federal, state, and local governments is expected to increase by 2 percentage points over the projection period, reaching 47 percent by 2027.
- The insured share of the population is expected to remain stable at around 90 percent throughout 2018-27 (CMS, National Health Expenditure Data: Projections, 2019).

International Comparisons, 1970-2019

- Relative to the size of its wealth, the U.S. spends a disproportionate amount on healthcare . As would be expected, wealthy countries like the U.S., tend to spend more per person on healthcare and related expenses than lower income countries. However, even as a high income country, the U.S. spends more per person on health than comparable countries.
- On average, other wealthy countries spend about half as much per person on health than the U.S. spends. Comparing health spending in the U.S. to other countries is complicated, as each country has unique political, economic, and social attributes that contribute to its spending. Because health spending is closely associated with a country's wealth, the remaining charts compare the U.S. to similar OECD countries –those that have above median national incomes (as measured by GDP) and also have above median income per person.

- Since 1980, the gap has widened between U.S. health spending and that of other countries. Over the past four decades, the difference between health spending as a share of the economy in the U.S. and comparable OECD countries has widened.
- While the U.S. has similar public spending on health, its private sector spending is triple that of comparable countries. While the U.S. has much higher total spending as a share of its economy, its public expenditures alone are in line with other countries. In 2016, the U.S. spent about 8.5 percent of its GDP on health out of public funds –essentially equivalent to the average of the other comparable countries. However, private spending in the U.S. is much higher than any comparable country; 8.8 percent of GDP in the U.S., compared to 2.7 percent on average for other nations.
- The U.S. has increased both public and private sector spending at a faster rate than similar countries. Over the last three decades, healthcare spending in the U.S. has increased in both the public and private sectors. Comparable countries increased private sector spending from 1.4 percent to 2.7 percent of GDP from 1970 to 2017, while the U.S. increased private sector spending from 3.9 percent to 8.8 percent during the same period. In 2017, the U.S. spent around 8.5 percent of GDP on health through public funds, a rate similar to comparable countries (Sawyer and Cox, 2018, Figures 1-7).

A FACTS-BASED CRITICAL ASSESSMENT

Healthcare in the United States is provided by many distinct organizations. Healthcare facilities are largely owned and operated by private sector businesses. Fifty eight percent of community hospitals are non-profit, 21 percent are government owned, and 21 percent are for-profit. "Adoption of single payer national health system (replacing for-profit private insurers) would significantly reduce the resources devoted to unusual ways of paying for healthcare. It would eliminate the private insurance sector's participation, reduce employers' costs of administering healthcare plans, reduce the costs incurred by doctors and hospitals due to billing insurers as well as pursuing patients for uncovered cost, lower the costs of appealing denials, and cut costs associated with patients avoiding early treatment of diseases (because of the actual or expected out-of-pocket costs) that become chronic and expensive maladies" (Nersisyan & Wray, 2019, p. 26; U.S. Census Bureau, New 2018 Service Annual Survey Data Released).

The health of the population is also viewed as a measure of the overall effectiveness of the healthcare system. The extent to which the population lives longer healthier lives signals an effective system and significantly contributes to a healthier human capital. Yet, a concern for the health system is that the health gains do not accrue uniformly to the entire population. Those who are insured may be underinsured because they cannot afford adequate medical care. In practice, the uninsured are often treated, but the cost is covered through taxes and other fees which shift the cost. Forgone medical care due to extensive cost sharing may ultimately increase costs due to downstream medical issues; this dynamic may be one factor to high healthcare expenditures in the U.S. when compared to other countries.

From a macroeconomic standpoint, "while the distribution of spending between private and public sectors would change, causing a lot of anxiety about potentially ballooning government deficits, there is nothing about government spending that necessarily makes it more inflationary than private spending –all else equal". Indeed, according to estimates by Nersisyan and Wray (2019), Medicare-for-all "could save from 2.61 percent to 3.67 percent of GDP, depending on the assumptions, while providing healthcare to the whole population" (p. 30). Consequently, "if private spending on healthcare costs falls by more than the increased spending by [Federal] government, the movement to single payer will be deflationary, not inflationary" (Ibid., p. 31). Others predict savings of about 1.58 percent of GDP (Pollin et al., 2018, p. 27). "What will really matter is the overall increase of demand on resources" while implementing a national health and insurance scheme and, perhaps, focusing more on preventive medicine (Nersisyan & Wray, 2019, p. 27).

Moreover, a large demographic shift in the United States is putting pressure on the medical system as "baby boomers" reach retirement age. The demographic shift to an older population is projected to increase medical spending in the United States by at least 5 percent, creating a funding challenge that the government (through Medicare and other social services), insurance companies, and individual savings accounts will strain to absorb. Evidently, the older population is rapidly increasing demand for healthcare services despite the tight budgets and reduced workforce. All of these factors put pressure on wages and working conditions, with some healthcare jobs seeing salary reductions (Papanicolas, Woskie, & Jha, 2018).

SUGGESTIONS FOR A COMPREHENSIVE NATIONAL HEALTH SYSTEM

It is our opinion that everyone should be included in a single public plan covering all medically necessary services, including acute, rehabilitative, long-term, and home care; mental health services; dental services; occupational healthcare ; prescription drugs and medical supplies; and preventive and public health measures. Boards of experts and community representatives would determine which services were unnecessary or ineffective, and these would be excluded from coverage. As in Canada, alternative insurance coverage for services included under the national health program would be eliminated, as would patient copayments and deductibles. Whether a universal health and insurance coverage scheme enhances economic growth or productivity or contributes to a more fair and better society depends on how such a national health program is constructed and which services are particularly emphasized given that a just society takes care of such basic social needs.

Clearly, the "Medicare-for-all" proposal is completely different from the Certificate of Need (CON) that many States have. Although there is a large degree of variation between different States, CON laws are basically designed to control the growth and associated costs of healthcare facilities and services, coordinate the planning of healthcare facilities, and avoid duplication (Kagan, 2018). Universal coverage would solve the crucial problem in healthcare by eliminating financial barriers to care. Considering existing health disparities in the U.S., a single comprehensive program is necessary both to ensure equal access to care and to minimize the complexity and expense of billing and administration. The public administration of insurance funds would save tens of billions of dollars each year.

The complexity of the current insurance system, with its multiplicity of payers, forces U.S. hospitals to spend more than twice as much as Canadian hospitals on billing and administration and requires U.S. physicians to spend about 10 percent of their gross incomes on excess billing costs (OECD, 2019). Eliminating insurance programs that duplicated the national health program coverage, though politically thorny, would clearly be within the prerogative of the U.S. Federal government. Failure to do so would require continuation of the costly bureaucracy necessary to administer and deal with such a program (Pollin at al., 2018; Nersisyan & Wray, 2019).

Copayments and deductibles endanger the health of poor people who are sick, decrease the use of vital inpatient medical services as much as they discourage the use of unnecessary ones, discourage preventive care, and are unwieldy and expensive to administer. Canada has few such charges, yet health costs are lower than in the United States and have risen more slowly. In the United States, in contrast, increasing copayments and deductibles have failed to slow the escalation of costs. Instead of the confused and often unjust dictates of insurance companies, a greatly expanded program of technology assessment and cost-effectiveness evaluation would guide decisions about covered services, as well as about the allocation of funds for capital spending, drug formularies, and other issues (OECD, 2019; Papanicolas, Woskie, & Jha, 2018).

Current capital spending greatly affects future operating costs as well as the distribution of resources. Effective health planning requires that funds go to high-quality, efficient programs in the areas of greatest need. Under the existing reimbursement system, which combines operating and capital payments, prosperous hospitals can expand and modernize, whereas impoverished ones cannot, regardless of the health needs of the population they serve or the quality of services they provide. The national health program would replace this implicit mechanism for distributing capital with an explicit one, which would facilitate allocation on the basis of need and quality. Insulating these crucial decisions from distortion by narrow interests would require the rigorous evaluation of the technology and assessment of needs, as well as the active involvement of providers and patients (Nersisyan & Wray, 2019).

Undoubtedly, such an alternative health policy framework would need a different public finance viewpoint at the federal and state levels. Still, funds for the construction or renovation of health facilities and for purchases of major equipment would be appropriated from the national health program budget. The funds would be distributed by state and regional health-planning boards composed of both experts and community representatives. Capital projects funded by private donations would require approval by the health-planning board if they entailed an increase in future operating expenses. The national health program would pay owners of for-profit hospitals, nursing homes, and clinics a reasonable fixed rate of return on existing equity. Since virtually all new capital investment would be funded by the national health program, it would not be included in calculating the return on equity (Nersisyan & Wray, 2019).

In short, the healthcare system of the United States is failing. Tens of millions of people are uninsured, costs are skyrocketing, and the bureaucracy is expanding. The federal government has the important responsibility to support adequate social services and promote the well-being of citizens. Reforms can only succeed in exchanging old problems for socially-sensitive solutions. What is being emphasized here is a national health program that would 1. fully cover everyone under a single, comprehensive public insurance program; 2. pay hospitals and nursing homes a total annual amount to cover all operating expenses; 3. fund capital costs through separate appropriations; 4. pay for physicians services and ambulatory services in any of three ways: through fee-for-service payments with a simplified fee schedule and mandatory acceptance of the national health program payment as the total payment for a service or procedure (assignment), through budgets for hospitals and clinics employing salaried physicians, or on a *per capita* basis (fee); 5. be funded, at least initially, from the same sources as at present, but with payments disbursed from a single pool; and 6. contain costs through savings on bureaucracy and billing, improved proficient health planning, and the ability of the national health program as the single payer for services to establish overall spending limits.

CONCLUSION

As expected, the chapter leaves many puzzling problems unsolved. Much detailed preparation would be needed to ease dislocations during the implementation of a Medicare-for-all program. Neither the encouragement of preventive healthcare and healthful lifestyles nor improvements in occupational and environmental health would automatically follow from the institution of a national health program. Similarly, racial, linguistic, geographic, and other nonfinancial barriers to access would persist. The need for continuing to fund higher education for healthcare providers in times of shortage would be no less pressing. Establishing research priorities and directing funds to high-quality investigations would be no easier. Further work in the area of long-term care would be required. Regional health planning and capital allocation would make possible, but not ensure, the fair and efficient allocation of resources. Finally, although all these problems would not be solved, a comprehensive national health program would establish a framework for addressing them.

Through this chapter, assuming that modern forms of intervention ought to be socially sensitive and egalitarian (given the range and magnitude of health problems in the United States), we seek to provide a realistic framework for genuine public debate of fundamental health policy requirements. A national health and insurance scheme or a universal Medicare-for-all will undoubtedly encounter powerful opponents in the health insurance industry, firms that do not now provide health benefits to employees, and medical entrepreneurs. There are also allies. For instance, most physicians (56 percent) support a single-payer health system, and about half (49 percent) support Medicare-for-all (Bluth, 2017; Finnegan, 2019). Many of the largest corporations would enjoy substantial savings if such a proposal were adopted. More significantly, the great majority of Americans would greatly benefit from a universal, comprehensive, publicly administered national health system. If properly mobilized, public confidence can override even the most strenuous private and political opposition and lobbyism. Most importantly, a sophisticated understanding of the needs for socially sensitive government action is required to appropriate selection of thorough, technically proficient, and well-planned healthcare strategies and policies.

REFERENCES

Anderson, G. F., Hussey, P. & Petrosyan, V. (2019). It's still the prices, stupid: Why the US spends so much on healthcare, and a tribute to Uwe Reinhardt. *Health Affairs, 38*(1), 87-95, January. https://doi:10.1377/hlthaff.2018.05144

Anderson, G. F., Hussey, P. and Petrosyan, V. (2013). It's the prices, stupid: Why the United States is so different from other countries?. *Health Affairs, 22*(3), 89-105, May-June. doi:10.1377/hlthaff.22.3.89

Bluth, R. (2017). Doctors warm to single-payer healthcare. *Kaiser Health News*. https://khn.org/news/doctors-warm-to-single-payer-health-care/

Bond, J. R., & Smith, K. B. (2016). *Analyzing American democracy: Politics and political science* (2nd ed.). Routledge. doi:10.4324/9781315648538

Finnegan, J. (2019). Poll finds 49% of doctors support 'Medicare-for-All'. *FierceHealthcare*. https://www.fiercehealthcare.com/practices/poll-finds-49-doctors-support-medicare-for-all

Gallup (2020). Personal health issues. *Gallup*. https://news.gallup.com/poll/1648/personal-health-issues.aspx

Kagan, J. (2018). Certificate of Need. Health Insurance Basics. *Investopedia*. https://www.investopedia.com/terms/c/certificate-of-need.asp

Keynes, J. M. (1940). *How to pay for the war: A radical plan for the Chancellor of the Exchequer*. Macmillan.

Nersisyan, Y., & Wray, L. R. (2019). How to pay for the Green New Deal. *Working Paper No. 931*. Levy Economics Institute of Bard College.

Papanicolas, I., Woskie, L. R. and Jha, A. K. (2018). Healthcare spending in the United States and other high-income countries. *Clinical Review & Education, 319*(10), 1024-1039. https://doi:10.1001/jama.2018.1150

Pollin, R., Heintz, J., Arno, P., Wicks-Lim, J., & Ash, M. (2018). *Economic analysis of Medicare-for-All, November 30*. Political Economy Research Institute.

Richardson, C. R. (2011). Mandatory health insurance: Lessons from Massachusetts. In J. M. Bailey, C. Chin-Loy, N. Karagiannis, & Z. Madjd-Sadjadi (Eds.), *Modern competitiveness in the twenty-first century: Global experiences* (pp. 93–104). Lexington Books.

Sawyer, B., & Cox, C. (2018). How does health spending in the U.S. compare to other Countries? Peterson-KFF. *Health System Tracker*. https://www.healthsystemtracker.org/chart-collection/health-spending-u-s-compare-countries/#item-start

Schuck, P. H., & Wilson, J. Q. (Eds.). (2008). *Understanding America: The anatomy of an exceptional nation*. Public Affairs Books.

U.S. Census Bureau. (2018). Health insurance coverage in the United States: 2017. *Report No. P60-264*. U.S. Census Bureau.

OECD. (2018). OECD health statistics. [Data set]. https://www.oecd-ilibrary.org/social-issues-migration-health/data/oecd-health-statistics_health-data-en

TPC. (2022). *Briefing Book.* Urban Institute and Brookings Instution. https://www.taxpolicycenter.org/briefing-book/what-are-sources-revenue-federal-government

Center on Budger and Policy Priorities. (2022). Policy Basics: Where do federal tax revenues come from? *CBPP*. https://www.cbpp.org/research/federal-tax/policy-basics-where-do-federal-tax-revenues-come-from

DATA SOURCES

CBO. (2022). *Healthcare.* [Data set.] https://www.cbo.gov/topics/health-care

CDC. (2022). *Table 42*. [Data set]. https://www.cdc.gov/nchs/data/hus/2018/042.pdf

CDC. (2022). *Table 43*. [Data set]. https://www.cdc.gov/nchs/data/hus/2018/043.pdf

CMS. (2022). *NHE Fact Sheet.* [Data set]. https://www.cms.gov/research-statistics-data-and-systems/statistics-trends-and-reports/nationalhealthexpenddata/nhe-fact-sheet

CMS. (2022). *National Health Care Spending in 2016.* [Data set]. https://www.cms.gov/Research-Statistics-Data-and-Systems/Statistics-Trends-and-Reports/NationalHealthExpendData/Downloads/NHE-Presentation-Slides.pdf

Blog, H. H. (2022). *Harvard Health Publishing*. [Data set]. https://www.health.harvard.edu/blog/

Health Care Facts. (2022). Healthcare in America costs too much. [Data set].

https://www.healthcarefacts.info/?utm_source=pm_search&utm_content=C4&gclid=EAIaIQobChMIgYO16fP55QIVA-iGCh05xwAnEAAYASAAEgKOOfD_BwE

U.S. Census Bureau. (2022). *Current Population Survey (CPS) – Annual Social and Economic Supplements (ASEC) and the American Community Survey (ACS).* [Data set]. https://www.census.gov/topics/health.html

U.S. Census Bureau. (2022). *Health.* [Data set]. https://www.census.gov/topics/health/data.html

U.S. Census Bureau. (2022). *Health Data.* [Data set]. https://www.census.gov/programs-surveys/cps/data-detail.html

Statista. (2022). *National per capita health since 1960.* [Data set]. https://www.statista.com/statistics/184955/us-national-health-expenditures-per-capita-since-1960/

OECD. (2020). *Life expectancy at birth.* [Data set]. https://data.oecd.org/healthstat/life-expectancy-at-birth.htm

OECD. (2019). OECD health statistics 2019. [Data set]. https://www.oecd.org/els/health-systems/health-data.htm

APPENDIX

Figure 1. US healthcare spending as a share of GDP

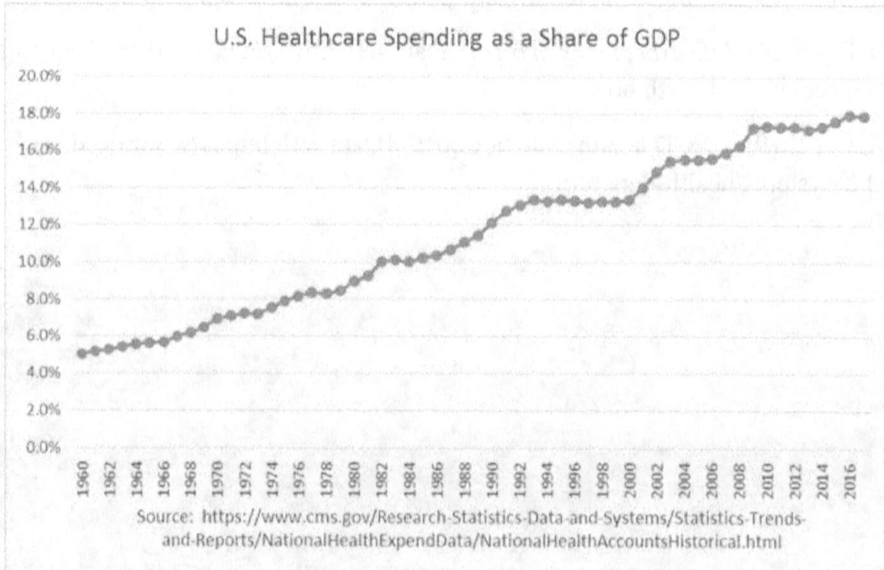

Figure 2. Number of federal and nonfederal hospitals in the US from 1975 to 2017

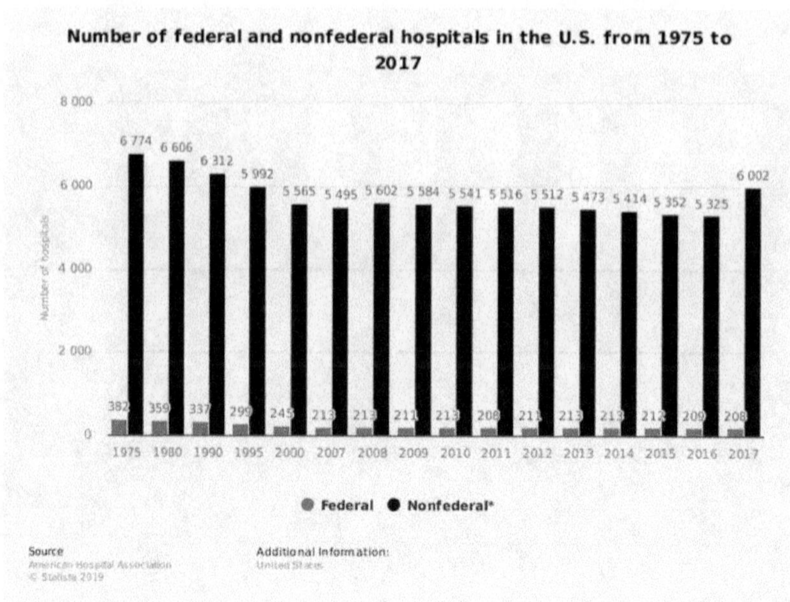

Chapter 4
What Can Economics Tell Us About What Is Right and Wrong With Our Healthcare System?

Zagros Madjd-Sadjadi
Winston-Salem State University, USA

Enrico Marcelli
San Diego State University, USA

ABSTRACT

This chapter describes the difference between health and health care, the efficacy and efficiency of the US health care system, the institutional framework of the US healthcare system, and the positive and negative features of the system, as well as recommendations for change. The authors note that US healthcare is both among the world's best and the developed world's worst, depending on what is being used as a basis for comparison. The complexity of the system with its seven different methods of payment is taken to task, and the fact that health care is an industry that significantly deviates from classical economic industrial theory is evaluated in depth. It is noted that economics can tell us much about how the misaligned and inappropriate incentives, as well as the erroneous comparisons to other industries, have allowed politicians to mislead the public as to the true benefits and drawbacks of the US health care system, which is better described as "sick care" as opposed to "health care."

DOI: 10.4018/978-1-6684-4060-5.ch004

INTRODUCTION

It is the best of systems, it is the worst of systems, it has the best doctors, it has the worst access, it has the best medical care in the world, it has the worst obesity rate in the world, it writes off more medical care for the uninsured in the world, it has the highest rate of medical debt bankruptcy in the world, its medical advances are unrivaled, its healthcare disparities are unrivaled, some have more choices for care than anywhere else, some have fewer choices for care than anywhere else, we have private medicine, we have socialized medicine – in short, the current medical system in the United States is so unlike that found in other locales, that some of the loudest critics and greatest supporters can find in the data surrounding our system whatever comparison they wish to make. This parody of Charles Dickens' opening line to *A Tale of Two Cities* is reminiscent of the state of American healthcare today as seen through the lenses of both liberals and conservatives depending on their ideological bent.

This chapter will consist of six sections following this introduction. The first will discuss the difference between health and healthcare because these are often misunderstood concepts that are often conflated in discussion of the efficacy and efficiency of the US healthcare system. In the second, we will discuss the institutional framework of the healthcare system in the United States. The third will discuss the positive features of the US healthcare system. The fourth will provide drawbacks and this is followed by recommendations for changes to the current system. A conclusion rounds out this chapter.

HEALTH OR HEALTHCARE?

We should begin by differentiating between health and healthcare as well as how economists view health as opposed to the medical profession. If you look at a standard definition of health, such as that as defined by the World Health Organization (1946), it "is a state of complete physical, mental and social well-being and not merely the absence of disease or infirmity." However, economists define health as a durable good, a form of human capital, that allows individuals to create services over the individual's lifetime based on the composition of the stock of health capital (Grossman 1972a, 1972b). Effectively, one's health, at any given point in time, is a stock of capital that can be added to through better nutrition, exercise, and other investments, such as medical care, and that depreciates over time as we age if we do not replenish it. This depreciation accelerates as we age and eventually results in death when the stock of health capital becomes too low to sustain us. Our initial endowment of health capital is primarily determined by genetics and our parent's living conditions when we are born. Thus parents who have access to greater resources through insurance or initial wealth can overcome genetic defects in their children's initial allotment to a much greater extent than parents who lack access to such resources. As we age, our decisions, our environment, the decisions of those around us, and our access to other resources affect our ability to sustain or improve our health.

Unfortunately, while there are many different things that affect a person's health, access to healthcare is actually one of the least important. Of much greater significance are the genetic makeup of the individual, the socioeconomic landscape in which they live, and the day-to-day decisions that individuals make that have an impact on their health. Healthcare is a derived demand since few people seek healthcare for its own sake. Instead, they seek healthcare because their own health is failing, and they often fail to realize the impact their decisions have on their overall health because many of our decisions focus on the here-and-now while one's need for healthcare is postponed to some future period.

We all know of the person who smokes cigars, eats poorly, and yet lives to a ripe old age with apparently little infirmity and we also know of people who take abundant care of themselves and yet succumb to a crippling disease or injury far earlier than they ought if life were fair, which it is not. We must understand that any type of discussion on healthcare needs to come back to this fundamental point, it is not because of a lack of spending on healthcare that we are unhealthy as a nation. Indeed, healthcare expenditures are 17.7% of our GDP, or more than 1 out of every 6 dollars in this economy, and have consumed an ever-greater share of GDP over the years (Martin et al., 2020).

According to the Global World Health Database of the World Health Organization, only two countries in the world spend more on healthcare as a percentage of their GDP than the United States. These are the micronations of Tuvalu and the Marshall Islands. Tuvalu has a population of 11,448 and the Marshall Islands has a population of 78,831 (CIA World Factbook 2021). If we exclude nations with populations of less than 250,000 as well as low-income or low-middle income countries, we find the United States spends significantly more on healthcare both as a percentage of GDP and in per capita terms purchasing power parity terms than any other country (see Tables 1, 2).

Given how much we spend on healthcare, it would be reasonable to expect the US has the best outcomes when it comes to life expectancy. Unfortunately, while every single country on the purchasing power parity list had an average life expectancy at birth of at least 81.3 years in 2019, the United States has a life expectancy of only 78.5 years in that same year. The US ranked *40th* in the world in life expectancy behind such countries as Turkey, Croatia, Estonia, Panama, Costa Rica, Slovenia, and Kuwait, none of which spend anywhere close to what the US spends on healthcare on either a per capita or percentage of GDP basis (World Health Organization 2021b).

Among all countries in the first table, the only ones that do worse in life expectancy are Cuba, Argentina, Armenia, and Brazil, all of which are much poorer countries. Perhaps we do better in terms of healthy life expectancy? After all, who wants to be infirm in one's old age? Unfortunately, we do even worse here, dropping to 68th place with an abysmal 66.1 years of health lifespan, while those living in every other country in the list in Table 2 have at least 4 more years of healthy lives than US residents do. Indeed, people living in Iran, Jamaica, Algeria, Serbia, Cuba, and China all live longer in terms of healthy lives than do Americans (World Health Organization 2021b).

Table 1. Percentage of GDP spent per capita (2018) on healthcare consumption

Country	% of GDP
United States of America	16.9%
Switzerland	11.9%
Germany	11.4%
France	11.3%
Cuba	11.2%
Japan	11.0%
Sweden	10.9%
Canada	10.8%
Austria	10.3%
Belgium	10.3%
Denmark	10.1%
Norway	10.0%
Armenia	10.0%
United Kingdom	10.0%
Netherlands	10.0%
Argentina	9.6%
Brazil	9.5%
Maldives	9.4%
Portugal	9.4%
Australia	9.3%
Source: World Health Organization 2021a)	

Table 2. Per capita expenditure on healthcare based on purchasing power parity (2018)

Country	US$ PPP
United States of America	$10,624
Switzerland	$8,114
Norway	$6,818
Germany	$6,098
Luxembourg	$6,048
Ireland	$5,897
Austria	$5,879
Sweden	$5,828
Denmark	$5,794
Netherlands	$5,635
Belgium	$5,405
France	$5,250
Canada	$5,200
Iceland	$5,113
Australia	$5,005
United Kingdom	$4,620
Japan	$4,504
Finland	$4,457
Singapore	$4,439
New Zealand	$4,024
Malta	$3,897
Source: World Health Organization (2021a)	

So what about our elderly? Surely they do better. After all, we have universal medical coverage with Medicare to help them. However, it turns out that we do not do much better with our elderly population. When we turn to life expectancy numbers for those at age 60, we find that we rank 37th in the world and when we examine healthy life spans, we are tied for 49th with Brazil, El Salvador, and Jamaica with an average of 16.4 years of healthy life spans remaining, while top-rated Japan's residents can count on 4 additional healthy years to live (World Health Organization 2021b).

It gets even worse. US life expectancy has been plunging due to the coronavirus. In the first six months of 2020, US life expectancy dropped by a full year over the comparable period in 2019, while life expectancy among African-Americans declined by 2.7 years and among Hispanic-Americans, life expectancy reduced by

1.9 years (Thompson 2021). This is anomalous compared to other countries since the US death rate per million people due to Coronavirus is the eighth highest in the world behind only Czechia, Belgium, Slovenia, the UK, Italy, Portugal, and Hungary (Statista 2021). This death rate is also more concerning because of the fact that the US has spent more on the coronavirus response as a percentage of GDP than all but Japan, Slovenia, Sweden, Finland, and Germany (Barone 2020).

INSTITUTIONAL FRAMEWORK

The US healthcare system is really not one system but a variety of systems that form a complex web of interactions. This leads to strange results. Since healthcare is intangible in that it is very difficult for patients to assess its efficacy, there is a lot of information asymmetry between provider and patient. This makes it difficult for individuals to be able to properly assess the quality of healthcare that they receive. In addition, most individuals have insurance of one form or another that pays a substantial portion of the cost of healthcare and most doctor's offices and hospitals fail to provide any type of price transparency when it comes to provision of services. Healthcare is the only commodity that is provided up front with no knowledge of how much the eventual cost to the consumer will be, yet it is simultaneously the most expensive expenditures on a cumulative basis that individuals will make. When it comes to economics, this is a problem. Standard economic modeling assumes the following in order to derive its conclusions that the free market is the best solution:

(1) Perfect information about quality
(2) Perfect information about prices
(3) Consumers are rational in making purchases
(4) Entry and exit from the market is relatively easy
(5) There are large numbers of firms and consumers, each having little or no effect on market prices
(6) All firms sell identical products
(7) There is no government regulation or at least none that benefits one group at the expense of another so as to unbalance the market.

All of these assumptions are violated by the healthcare industry to some degree depending on the industry and the institutional framework we are examining. When one or more of these assumptions is violated, not only is the free market no longer necessarily the best solution but it might not even be the most efficient solution (Wolf, Jr. 1988). Indeed, we could almost say that healthcare has become inefficient by design. After all, "healthcare in the United States in extraordinarily inefficient" and in the generational period between 1990 and 2011, its productivity actually declined by 0.9% *per year* while the rest of the economy gained in productivity by 2.2% per year, meaning "healthcare has become less inefficient as the overall economy has become more efficient" (Wenz 2015: 161). The functional purpose of all of this is "to support many jobs and increase one corporate profits" and if we were to cut back on the level of healthcare spending in this country to even a level more in line with the second highest expender on healthcare as a percentage of GDP among all industrialized countries (Canada), over 5 million people would lose their jobs (Wenz 2015: 188). So while generating more efficiencies and reducing the cost of healthcare might seem to be good tradeoff in the theoretical sphere, it must be noted that many of these individuals would need extensive retraining to enter other fields of work and this retraining means that the efficiency returns we would realize by reducing our costs would be offset by the retooling costs. This is not an argument against making rather draconian cost cutting in the healthcare sector because the current system is simply unsustainable but it points to a political reality – the healthcare industry will not go down without a fight.

This is particularly problematic when one looks at why healthcare is so inefficient. Any substantially labor-intensive process will often have significant productivity inefficiencies. There is a reason why the world's population in 1700 AD had approximately the same productivity as they did in 1700 BC: productivity is predominantly enhanced through one of five processes: (1) more capital per worker; (2) better technology; (3) better management; (4) better worker skill; or (5) scale economies with rising output (Heilbrun 2013) As such, when industries are labor intensive and the output is measured by simply the hours worked, such as is the case in healthcare, it is extraordinarily difficult to find measurable improvements in productivity. One 15-minute appointment with a patient with respect to a clinician's, therapist's, or nurse's time is going to always take the same amount of time regardless of improvements in technology. The only real hope is to reduce that amount of time somehow through an automated process such as using artificial intelligence so that the same information can be communicated in less than 15 minutes or so that the same 15 minutes can be devoted to multiple patients. This is how productivity improvements have occurred in the arts or education – by having larger performance or lecture halls, a performer or an educator can now serve more people in the same amount of time. However, healthcare does not allow for this to occur, so another method must be employed.

One way to improve provider productivity is to transfer the responsibility of care back to the patients by making them fill out detailed medical histories each and every time and fill out all possible complaints in advance. This reduces the amount of time spent with each patient. However, this is highly problematic to patients because they must fill out the same exact information each and every time and the non-standardized forms can make it difficult for them to provide an accurate accounting. When we combine this with a lack of a centralized health database, the opportunity for errors to creep in skyrockets. It is estimated that 70% of all health records contain errors, a completely unacceptable amount given the critical need for proper information (Spitzer 2018). The amount of time undertaken by doctors will be lessened but this is usually because of an increase in the time spent by patients up front. When patients have low or no co-pays, they will likely find this tradeoff offensive. After all, the tradeoff is to require the patients to spend time that the doctor does not have to spend but the patient was never paying for the true cost of the doctor's time at the time of the appointment. While this may lower overall healthcare costs, patients will not believe this to be the case at the margin and thus might object.

To combat this, we could create a system where electronic medical record bureaus act similar to credit reporting bureaus that aggregate all medical records but then the medical records would be sent to each patient, who would own the medical records and be given an opportunity to point out and have critical errors corrected. When a patient comes in for medical care, there would be an automatic pulling of the medical records for each patient from the major medical reporting bureaus. When aggregated, such a system would ideally operate in the exact opposite way as we see occur with combined credit reports whereby the only information that will be allowed in would be information that is consistent across all medical reporting bureaus. That way if errors creep in at one bureau they will be kept off the aggregated report unless all of the bureaus have the exact same information (Richardson, Hall, and Madjd-Sadjadi 2010). The problem is that patients are often blamed for errors that come about in the coding process and the only times they are believed is when the statement is clearly false. One of the authors has a good friend who found out that his medical report said that he was being treated for uterine cancer, which was quite a shock to say the least given that he is, and has always been, male. Additionally, it can be very costly both in terms of money but also in terms of health outcomes, to be running additional tests simply because the current doctor did not order it. Many medical tests, such as x-rays and CT scans, have non-negligible risks if they are repeated unnecessarily. This is why each patient, not the medical providers, needs to be in charge of his or her own medical records.

Another possibility is to use artificial intelligence to make the patient effectively self-diagnose. However, this can be dangerous as well. By providing automated tools in the hands-on non-experts, there is the distinct possibility of misdiagnosis not unlike what we see with what is known as the WebMD effect whereby the increased availability of healthcare information has caused rampant self-misdiagnosis. Indeed, upwards of 75% of Americans report using MD to provide medical advice and 60% of Americans due it each month. The problem is that when non-experts search these well-meaning databases, they often come to the worst possible conclusion about their actual conditions rather than the most likely conclusion, which is that they should not worry at all (Brownell 2011). If we give non-experts these tools, they could end up running even more often to the doctor than they already do. Of course, if these tools are used exclusively by doctors and other medical personnel, it can serve to lower costs. However, at the end of the day, patients expect to see doctors and while they "do not care how much labor is used as an input into the production of a car, [...] they do care how much labor input is used in a massage, artistic performance, or doctor's visit. It is hard to increase labor productivity if what is being purchased is the time and attention of the laborer." (Helland and Tabarrok 2019, 41-42)

Going back to our seven assumptions about a free market, it should be noted that at least one of these assumptions is violated in every healthcare sector and in some cases, such as emergency room visits when patients are unconscious, *all* of them are violated. In some cases, such as eyeglasses, all of these assumptions *appear* to be met. Most opticians and optometrists post prices for everyone to see, consumers tend to understand what it means to be farsighted or nearsighted, it is relatively easy to enter the eyeglasses marketplace, prescription lenses are standardized, and there is little in the way of government regulation compared to other healthcare areas. However, there is more than meets the eye. For example, one company, Luxottica, has an outsized impact on the industry for eyeglass frames. It owns several chains of what would appear at first glance to be competing eyeglass stores such as Lenscrafters, Oliver Peoples, and Pearle Vision. It owns outright Oakley and Ray-ban and licenses frames for sale for Chanel, Giorgio Armani, and Prada, among others. It owns the second largest vision care insurer, EyeMed. While there is considerable competition from independent optometrists, Costco, and Walmart, Luxottica also handles Target's glasses unit, Target Optical (Luxottica 2021).

It gets worse. The biggest problem is that our brains are hardwired for immediate and guaranteed satisfaction while the benefits from health tend to be more long-term and probabilistic. A low inflation rate ought to be enough to allow us to be more interested in our long-term prognosis since it reduces the discount rate by which we discount the future. However, inflation does not seem to be correlated with health outcomes predominantly because many people believe that they will not pay for these costs in their old age. Indeed, just 13% of all Americans have specifically set aside money to take care of healthcare costs despite the fact that healthcare costs are the single biggest expense in retirement and a whopping 26% actually think that government benefits will take care of all of their expenses (Bank of America 2020, p. 17). As such, we are decidedly not rational when it comes to making healthcare decisions.

While economics would suggest that one way to resolve this dilemma is to go to fee-for-service and eliminate insurance, this is not likely to be a good solution. Sticker shock would likely make seeing the doctor much less likely in many cases since we have established a form of path dependency where third-party payers are the norm, not the exception. Furthermore, it is unclear whether the healthcare industry itself would like to have greater price transparency. The current system is more akin to what we see in higher education where government programs are used to finance them. While much of the financial aid that is doled out is in the form of loan programs, these are often discounted by students who think of the cost as a form of "investment" even though they can get a high-quality education at a much cheaper price by going to public universities and eschewing private ones. Rather than setting a maximum loan disbursement at the level of in-state or even out-of-state tuition, students are encouraged to take on large amounts of debt to private schools and to even take on debt for ordinary living expenses. Fully 27% of all millennials did not understand the terms and conditions of the student loan programs for which they were signing (Hoffower 2020). Educational officials and politicians stress the desire to have students graduate "on time," meaning in a four-year period, rather than thinking about the need for students to plan their education in such a way as to limit loans by stretching their education over a longer period of time. Students, rather than going into excessive debt, should go to school part-time and work part-time but this sort of financial literacy is neither taught nor encouraged. This is further complicated when politicians in the interest of getting votes start to suggest that loan forgiveness ought to be on the table. This simply encourages people to go further into debt with the expectation that they will be bailed out later (Farrington 2019).

Yet there is a key difference between higher education and healthcare. Students entering into higher education see the sticker price of tuition, even if they ultimately ignore it. They often spend months determining which university to attend and have ample time to compare various financial aid packages before making a decision. However, "please take me to St. Joseph's Medical Center because they are having a 50% off sale on heart surgery this week" is something that no EMT has ever heard in the ambulance anywhere in the world when transporting someone with a heart attack. In emergency situations, it is possible that the person who is being taken to the emergency room is not even conscious and thus cannot actually contract for the services provided. It seems strange that we would allow a system to exist where people can be bankrupted because of someone else's decisions without regard to our own financial well-being.

There is another major difference between higher education and healthcare – there really is not one healthcare system in the United States, there are at least *seven*:

(1) a government-run healthcare system not unlike the UK's National Health System for veterans run by the Department of Veterans Affairs where the doctors and hospitals are employed by the government and care is coordinated by the government;

(2) a government-run federal insurance-based system for the elderly called Medicare;
(3) a system that is partially funded by the federal government but is run by individual state governments for the poor called Medicaid;
(4) an employment-based system where the employer selects an insurer or a group of insurers that employees may be able to select from;
(5) an individual purchase option where individual or small businesses purchase their own insurance directly from insurance companies without any subsidies;
(6) an individual purchase option that is subsidized by the government but where individuals purchase private insurance directly through the Health Insurance Marketplace® or by individual states that operate a similar service that was created by the Affordable Care Act (otherwise known as Obamacare); and
(7) a purely out-of-pocket system used primarily by the uninsured that often relies upon emergency room care but which is now expanding through companies such as FastMed that provide healthcare based on a fixed fee system.

Veterans Affairs

This is a single-payer, single-provider model where one entity, usually the government, provides all healthcare for the citizenry, often by using government-run clinics and provided by government-employed doctors, with little or no out-of-pocket costs incurred by the populace outside of taxes. This model on a national scale for all citizens was pioneered in the United Kingdom by William Beveridge and led to the creation of its National Health Service. In the United States, healthcare is provided for veterans through the Veterans Health Administration system of doctors at VA-owned medical centers, community living centers, and outpatient clinics. Some commentators (Chung 2017; Ebhomielen 2018) have noted that under the Beverage Model there can be long wait-times for "non-essential" services although the definition of "non-essential" is often a matter of debate since a hip replacement is certainly considered essential for those who are waiting to have one. However, a comparison between wait times at the Veterans' Administration between 2014 and 2017 by Penn et al. (2019), a period during which significant scrutiny and investments were made in the VA system due to public outcry over reports of long wait times, suggest that this is a function of funding rather than an inherent limitation of the model since new-appointment wait times were actually shorter than private sector wait times at the end of the reporting period.

Medicare

This is a single-payer, multiple-provider national model with the providers being private entities but costs are paid for by the federal government along with possible cost-sharing on the part of individuals. In the United States, this is most often seen a program used by individuals who are over the age of 65 or who have end-stage renal failure called Medicare.

Medicaid

This is a multiple-payer, multiple-provider state model with the providers being private entities but costs are paid out by states with assistance from the federal government. While Medicare eligibility and benefits are dictated by the federal government, the states have considerable leeway in determining these with Medicaid. Medicaid reimbursements for doctors are typically much lower than the rates are for Medicare and Medicaid often does not allow out-of-pocket charges for the very poor. In addition, the time to process reimbursements for Medicaid is often much longer than it is for Medicare (Mcaskill 2014). The combined state-federal system also means, not unlike what happens in Canada, there can be significant variation in terms of overall costs and experience from region to region that is much less present in a completely federalized system (Weil 2016). Since Medicaid is accepted by significantly fewer doctors than other payment methods, the fact that more than 1/3 of all working age African-Americans are on Medicaid, while only 1/6 of all European-Americans in the same age group are on it has potential implications for disparate health outcomes in medicine (Cohen et al., 2020).

Employment-based Insurance

Employment-based insurance is offered by 57% of all firms covering 90% of all workers (Hicks 2021). This is due to the fact that larger firms are the ones that are much more likely to provide such insurance than are the smallest of companies. Of course, being offered coverage does not mean that workers necessarily take it since such programs do allow for opting-out and often if one takes the insurance that is offered, there is a not insignificant premium attached to it. Employer-based insurance primarily arose in the United States during World War II after the War Labor Board ruled that fringe benefits were not subject to such wage and price controls that were imposed as part of the war effort to keep inflation and competition between firms in check (Buchmueller and Monheit 2009). Subsequent rulings by the National Labor Relations Board that allowed such benefits to be collectively bargained and by the Internal Revenue Service exempting premiums from income taxation made employer-provided health insurance only served to strengthen the link between employment and insurance. Large employers can reduce overall costs of insurance by spreading the risk across a larger group of individuals. For smaller employers, the lack of taxation can also it more beneficial to provide insurance than a similar amount of cash to employees to go purchase insurance on their own. This is because it will take a larger amount of money to fully compensation employees for the task of obtaining insurance on their own since monetary compensation is subject to income taxation while providing insurance is not. At the same time, because premiums are not subject to income taxation, the benefits from receiving employer-based insurance accrue more to high-income individuals than low-income individuals, providing a reverse Robin Hood effect whereby the poorer workers indirectly subsidize the richer workers. This is especially true when employers are self-insured and thus paying all the health insurance costs themselves, and can create a perverse incentive to allocate care on the basis of how valuable the employee is to the company. Individuals may choose to stay with companies longer than they would if insurance were not provided by employers, thus distorting labor market decisions, and it can lead to higher overall costs since federal and state governments are effectively subsidizing employer provision of such insurance through the income tax exemption of premiums.

Private Unsubsidized Insurance

For those who cannot get insurance from their employer or from the government program, there is the ability to purchase private unsubsidized insurance. Such purchases are somewhat problematic, though. Since insurance is based on risk, as individuals advance in age and decline in health status, their premiums tend to increase. This is unlike employer-based health insurance due to the pooling of risk across the entire organization, although if the pooled risk of all employees goes up, a similar, but somewhat muted, pattern still may emerge. Fairly few people participate in the unsubsidized market because such premiums are often paid for with after-tax income, averse selection causes people with low risk to avoid seeking health insurance, thus raising the risk profile for everyone else, and economies of scale are not present when purchasing health insurance outside of a group policy.

Obamacare/Affordable Care Act

To solve the problem of a lack of affordability of unsubsidized insurance, many low- and middle-income taxpayers who lack access to employer-based insurance may choose to obtain government-subsidized insurance through the Affordable Care Act's Health Insurance Marketplace®. The marketplace allows individuals to comparison shop between different plans at the bronze (60/40 plan), silver (70/30 plan), gold (80/20 plan), and platinum (90/10 plan). It enables them to use tax credits to help pay for insurance up front, and guarantee that they are receiving a set minimum standard of coverage (called essential health benefits) by the plan.

One can also purchase a catastrophic plan (also known as a major medical plan) that still covers the same essential services and has no-cost preventative services but it has extremely high deductibles. On the other hand, the deductible is the same as the maximum out-of-pocket cost after premiums.

No Insurance

The no insurance model is often described as being a problem within the American context but some people actually prefer it to the alternative. What needs to be understood is that while many Americans may find themselves with a lack of insurance due to a lack of affordable options, this is not always the case and it does not necessarily mean a lack of access to high quality medical care. High-income Americans may prefer to go without or may decide to spend outside of the insurance system simply because they can afford to do so. While Americans frequently hear that wealthy Canadians travel to the United States or other countries to receive medical care, Americans are actually nearly four times more likely to travel abroad for medical care than are Canadians with 0.41% of all Americans travelling abroad for medical care in comparison to just 0.11% of Canadians (Weil 2016: 357). The primary reason for this is cost – US medical care is significantly more expensive than healthcare in almost any other part of the world.

This is not universally true, however. Companies such as FastMed, which provides urgent care at a fixed cost that is prominently displayed when one enters the clinic, may help to reduce costs but if the individual lacks insurance as well as the ability to pay even a few hundred dollars for treatment, they very well might decide to forgo such clinics for the emergency room where they cannot be turned away due to an inability to pay (Yee, Lechner, and Boukus, 2013). Such a delay often must come at the cost of higher levels of criticality, which ends up increasing the costs of care for everyone as the charity care provided by the emergency rooms is passed on to insurance companies and the insured population. This type of free-riding occurs because emergency rooms are required by law to offer emergency medical care to everyone without regard to ability to pay while the US population is not required to have insurance or alternative means to pay for these medical bills. When there is an insignificant number of people in a society who lack such ability to pay, this free ridership will likely not be serious but when you have 14.7% of the working-age population and 29.7% of the Hispanic working age population lacking health insurance or sufficient assets to pay for medical treatment, this is going to be an issue (Cohen et al., 2020).

THE GOOD PARTS OF THE US HEALTHCARE SYSTEM

Perhaps the best aspect of the US healthcare system is maintaining its leadership in terms of research and development of new healthcare technologies. Nowhere in the world do we see the level of innovation that American firms have in terms of healthcare research and development. The United States in the world's largest exporter of Medical Instruments with 21.7% of all such trade (Observatory of Economic Complexity 2021). The US accounts for 40.6% of all biotechnology patents in the world, 68.3% of all life sciences venture capital in the OECD, 50.9% of all worldwide clinical trials, and the research and development of 40 of the world's top 75 best-selling medicine (DeVol el al. 2011: 5-6).

The general perception among the US public is that care, while unaffordable, is not rationed with the notable exception of organ transplants, for those who can pay for it based on lack of availability, a key complaint that is found in countries that have a larger role for government in their healthcare or health insurance provision. In addition, there appears to be significant clinician and patient autonomy, which is a direct result of the pay for service model adopted by most insurance companies (Luft 2006: 24).

According to the OECD (2021), despite significant barriers in terms of medical licensing, the United States has attracted over 215,000 foreign doctors representing 25% of all doctors in the country. In the case of every single OECD country except for New Zealand for which there is data on country of origin data for foreign doctors, there is a net brain drain from the country to the United States after considering the migration flows, both to and from the United States (See Table 3).

Unfortunately, healthcare utilization and quality statistics are not widely available for the US, so it is difficult to make meaningful comparisons between countries. However, when we look at two of the few statistics that is available, we find the United States does at least 20% more diagnostic exams per capita than any other OECD country and has the highest 5-year survival rate for breast cancer (OCED 2021).

We should also consider that the US system offers much more personalized care than any other system when it comes to individualized medical treatments. Only a society that allows the richest or most well insured among us to spend millions of dollars on their own care could achieve the successes in individualized treatments for diseases that only affect a handful of people or even just one. No broad-based medical care system could ever afford to spend millions upon millions of dollars to pay for one individual or to create a bloodline that eliminates whole categories of diseases due to individualized genomic treatments (Regalado 2018) or cancer treatments (Piore 2018).

Table 3. Doctor Brain Drain from OECD countries to US

	Doctors from US	Doctors to US	Net Brain Drain of Doctors
Australia	165	1187	*(1022)*
Austria	2	250	*(248)*
Belgium	96	729	*(633)*
Canada	1218	7765	*(6547)*
Chile	5	323	*(318)*
Czech Republic	0	547	*(547)*
Finland	15	45	*(30)*
France	7	645	*(638)*
Germany	243	2437	*(2194)*
Hungary	2	1059	*(1057)*
Israel	493	3483	*(2990)*
Italy	9	2270	*(2261)*
Netherlands	6	2870	*(2864)*
New Zealand	408	245	**163**
Norway	10	42	*(32)*
Poland	2	2833	*(2831)*
Portugal	7	75	*(68)*
Spain	71	1552	*(1481)*
Switzerland	86	369	*(283)*
Turkey	1	1337	*(1336)*
UK	70	4635	*(4565)*

The Bad Parts of the US Healthcare System

If these highly individualized treatment protocols using genetic screening and treatment sound suspiciously like eugenics with all of its intendant problems, that is because it is (Hercher 2018; Comfort 2018), though this is not based on race, perceived intelligence, or some other factor that inalienable quality but rather based on socioeconomic status. This plays into the overriding classist narrative that the poor somehow deserve to be poor due to some genetic predisposition or flawed character trait that pervades our uniquely puritanical set of beliefs. Treatments that excise genetic defeats may sound wonderful on the surface but threaten to create further health disparities among a society that already perceives itself as having the worst health disparities in the world based on how different income groups view the efficacy of the system (Hero, Zaslavsky, and Blendon 2017). When people believe that a system is fundamentally unfair, they are going to desire to change it.

More patient consultations (21.8%), medical tests (19.5%), and prescribed medicines (18.1%) were skipped due to costs in the US than in any other OECD country and the US has the fourth worst level of doctors leaving behind surgical items or device fragments in patient bodies after surgery, with only Canada, Sweden, and Australia performing worse on this metric (OECD 2021).

The US does not cover nearly as high of a percentage of its population through its insurance system as other countries, most of which have achieved near universal health insurance coverage. One of the major issues is that most Americans received their healthcare through their employers. While individual policies are available for purchase, they often are cost-prohibitive since group policies offered to companies often are lower-cost due to risk sharing within the enterprise. Employers negotiate with individual insurance companies for coverage for their employees and few offer coverage for retirees. Spouses and children insurance rates are often not subsidized by employers, making costs even higher for individuals who receive their insurance through their employer. Part-time employees and those who work for smaller companies often do not have any type of employer-based health insurance coverage. The employer-based system also tends to tie employees to the job since while employees are allowed to maintain their company's existing health insurance for a time, the employer subsidy for health insurance coverage is dropped once the person leaves employment with the company. There are additional issues as well: people are locked into the insurance based on what the employer chooses to negotiate. Rather than being able to freely choose from among a number of different insurance companies, such as is true for other types of insurance, the employer-based insurance model reduces consumer choice often to just a couple of policies offered by the same insurance company if there is any choice in the matter at all.

Every system of payment other than the no insurance model also suffers from the third-party payer problem that can lead to overconsumption of medical services. If I knew that the cost of a medical test is being covered by insurance, I might discount the cost and ask for it to go forward even if it provides little benefit from a cost-benefit analysis perspective. By shielding ourselves from the true cost of treatment, we also might be less likely to engage in behavioral changes that will positively impact our lives because the behavioral change costs exceed the out-of-pocket medical costs at the margin. For example, obesity is an incredibly serious health problem in the United States but inexpensive food coupled with inexpensive healthcare means that people are less likely to do something about this than if either of these were more expensive. On the other hand, because medical care comes with uncertainty, intertemporal externalities, and in some cases, consumption externalities (such as when we get vaccinated, we also protect others from the virus as well), a system that is based on user-pay only is likely to lead to underconsumption of certain medical services.

At the same time, the third party payer system suffers from defects as well. Bureaucratic systems can override patient care decisions in terms of whether to pay because the decision models cannot account for the complexities of individualized treatments. Patients may be treated by doctors who are out of network (a term used when the individual is seeking treatment at a provider who has not negotiated an agreement with the insurance company) even though the hospital they go to is in network. This can force individuals with insurance to incur substantial charges even though the patient may have had no means of knowing this in advance. Since mandatory coverage of healthcare services is regulated to a large extent at the state level, patients moving from one state to another can find themselves paying out of pocket for services for which they were insured in their original state.

Some individuals have a high deductible insurance plan and combine it with a Health Savings Account in what is known as a consumer directed healthcare plan. High deductibles and co-payments may discourage patients from seeking care early on when conditions are easier to treat (Luft 2016: 19) but the data on this is mixed with some arguing this is the case (Zhang, Trish, and Sood (2018) and others saying no (Haviland et al., 2016). There appears to be three reasons for these differences: two methodological and the other substantive. The first methodological issue is that we are more likely to come to a conclusion of yes when one uses a survey method because such studies often look at the issue from the standpoint of out-of-pocket expenditures without considering the premium savings that result from such plans or the fact that plan participants have access to a Health Savings Account to alleviate the burden. The second methodological issue is that we are more likely to come to a conclusion of no when we examine whether healthcare costs from the standpoint of insurer or employer records and look at overall costs or whether there are changes in the use of emergency rooms or hospitals as a proxy to determine whether the healthcare delay was proper or not. The issue is that such retrospective examination of data may not fully capture the criticality of delays in care because not all such delays may show up within the time frame under examination. The substantive issue is it appears as though this issue is predominantly found among those with lower incomes and who suffer from chronic conditions. Yet the tax preferential treatment and increased patient autonomy of these plans may conflict with the inherent self-interests of these populations. Those who have chronic conditions and those with lower incomes are often in a more vulnerable position to make care decisions on the basis of cost either because they may face liquidity constraints or they may be overly reliant on a doctor's advice for care, while healthier individuals are more likely to be able to make decisions based on financial outcomes (Bundorf 2016). Younger individuals, especially Millennials, who are generally less invested in traditional healthcare plan are also more likely to benefit from such plans (Beaton, 2017). One pervasive problem with them is that it is generally difficult for patients to determine what really is a high-value or a low-value healthcare service due to asymmetrical information between providers and patients. "Low-value medical services are medical tests and procedures that provide unclear or no clinical benefit to patients, but still expose them to both risk and expense" (Reid, Rabideau, and Sood 2017: 741) Unfortunately, there is little evidence that consumer directed health plans result in superior decision making in this regard (Reid, Rabideau, and Sood 2017). However, probably the harshest indictment against consumer directed healthcare is that the current medical system is just net set up and equipped to handle it. One of the authors spent months trying to correct a medical bill by trying to find the actual billing codes and then calling the insurance company and the provider's billing department to try to get each of them to see that the billing codes were inaccurate. There was no incentive on the part of either party to actually do the work to correct the error. The insurance company insisted that they could not tell the doctor what to code and the provider's billing department kept insisting that the code was correct. It was only after successfully talking to the doctor herself that the error was corrected. In another case, the same author had been prescribed a very expensive medicine by a doctor but the purpose of this medication was to treat an underlying condition that had no known symptoms and that was not necessarily malignant. After questioning this recommendation, the author decided against the treatment and has not had any of the averse reactions that the original doctor had anticipated would occur. These types of errors and issues are often only detected by an individual with an intimate knowledge of this field. Most people would simply unquestionably accept the advice of a doctor but if you do not understand what the doctor is ordering how can you possibly be an informed enough consumer to be able to properly take advantage of a consumer directed healthcare plan?

Another key issue is what is known as the certificate of need. The certificate of need requires that the potential entrant demonstrate that there is an actual need for the product, service, or procedure that is not currently being met by the market, not based on price but rather based on whether the product, service, or procedure is available in sufficient quantity to service all people in the market. This would be akin to having to a grocery store have to prove that there is an actual need for an addition grocery store, not based on price, but rather because people are unable to obtain food otherwise. All the existing grocery stores would need to do show that there was still food on their shelves and there would be no need established. In 36 states and the District of Columbia, healthcare expansion is limited in anywhere from one to 30 different markets. North Carolina, for example, regulates 25 different services, devices, or procedures. Vermont has the most such markets with 30 different ones, while Arizona regulates ground transport ambulance services (Koopman and

Stratmann 2015). This is despite the fact that general competition can never be a tort (Madjd-Sadjadi 2016; Friedman 1990). This does not mean that you cannot have competition torts, you definitely can, but these are not *a priori* restrictions on entry. They are instead restrictions on what you can in competition based on what is known as "unfair competition" but when "unfair competition" includes *all* competition, it should be manifestly obvious that, in this case, the restriction is illegitimate. To defend these actions, states argue that they are trying to reduce healthcare costs by limiting overinvestment. In addition, some states utilize a *quid pro quo* that requires providers who receive a certificate of need to provide charity care for poorer individuals, thus ensuring cross-subsidization occurs (Koopman and Stratmann 2015). However, neither of these arguments are cogent ones. Rather than charity care, governments can directly subsidize the poor in terms of healthcare, just as is the case with grocery stores, which do not receive a certificate of need to be established. As for the overinvestment argument, it also is a bad one since providers that are driven out of business will typically sell their equipment, thus ensuring that total investment is no greater in a competitive environment and it could be even less due to efficiencies that are introduced due to competitive pressures. Instead, it should be recognized that there is only one real point to the certificate of need system and that is to reduce price competition, which increases the elasticity of demand and thus *increases,* rather than decreases, healthcare costs. The true goal is to ensure that existing healthcare providers can maintain a market presence, helping to ensure they are guaranteed a profit even without having to compete with others, but a truly free market can never guarantee such a thing. Freedom to compete should never mean that everyone can succeed. Indeed, it should *always* mean that some will definitely fail. When you cannot fail, you cannot say that you succeeded.

RECOMMENDATIONS

There are many things we can do to strengthen existing coverage and extend coverage to uncovered or undercovered groups. One key factor is the elimination or dramatic reduction of traditional fee-for-service coverage. Part of the problem is that traditional fee-for-service provides the wrong incentive mechanisms. Rather than paying for health outcomes, you are paying for healthcare, which is not the same thing. This outcomes-based system is already in place but there can still be issues with it because you are still only incentivizing that which you are measuring. Areas that are difficult to measure, such as pain management or mental health, may receive even less attention than they do with traditional fee for service methods (Smith 1995). Just like with patients, doctors may choose to avoid the sickliest of patients for fear of losing the incentives that are given out (Mannion and Davies 2008). It is possible that there will be reductions in clinician autonomy but evidence suggests that this particular worry may be overblown (McDonald et al., 2007). One significant issue is that such incentive schemes need to be universal for them to be ineffective – if doctors face different incentives based on the insurer, the likelihood that they will be properly incentivized is reduced (Cutler 2004: 102). Pay for performance means that the doctor becomes responsible for the patient's well-being between office visits, not just at the time of consultation. It means following up with patients to ensure that they are taking their medications and are following through on proper treatments. This is already done with CPAP patients whose machines constantly monitor their use and can report back to doctors if they are not being used. It is also present in the drug Abilfy, which is used to treat schizophrenia, bipolar disorder, and depression. The drug has a sensor that syncs to a wearable patch that then transmits to a smart phone informing patients whether they have taken their drugs. The patient can then share this with their doctor (Fox 2017). Such measures, when they are in the control of patients, can lead to issues of moral hazard – patients who are not taking it are unlikely to report this to the doctor who cannot tell whether the patient who fails to report is taking the drug or not. In the case of CPAP machines, it can lead to individuals wearing the mask when they are not sleeping as the system may have difficulty distinguishing between whether a person is asleep or awake when using it. These types of "gaming the system" methods are present in most such incentive schemes. Wearing a smart watch to count steps can easily be gamed by merely shaking one's arm about. So long as there is a financial incentive, there will be the worry that people are not engaging in behavior that you want to see but rather the behavior you have incentivized.

Just because something is difficult to assess, it does not mean that it is impossible to assess. However, many people take the path of least resistance. Most pay for performance standards fail when we do not spend time to critically think about and understand exactly what we are incentivizing and whether there may be a superior way to accomplish this task. Incentivizing the wrong things can be incredibly detrimental but proper incentives can work wonders.

For example, to overcome the adverse selection problem, one can scale incentives based on what would be a value-added approach such that doctors are not compensated based solely on the outcomes but rather paid when they exceed the expected outcomes given the initial conditions. This type of system will ameliorate the adverse selection problem undertaken by providers and make it clear that we are paying for the marginal improvements created due to the provider's actions. This form of risk adjustment would go a long way towards alleviating such concerns (Cutler 2004: 110). One key benefit from this type of intervention is that an outcomes-based system avoids unnecessary regulations that can hamper patient and doctor autonomy. One persistent issue that comes to mind is that of opioids and marijuana, one of which has been handled correctly and the other, not so well. While limiting access to opioids is certain a noble goal, such limitations in a person with severe pain and facing end-of-life care would be an unnecessary and callous restriction, which is why both state and federal guidelines largely exempt such care from these limitations. Even still, we have the issue of medical marijuana that shows a lot of promise in helping with a wide variety of medical conditions but current federal law and many state laws prohibit access to it as a form of medicine. The point is that any blunt instrument that is based on punishment for deviance from its guidelines is prone to causing doctors to undertake incorrect treatment options. This is a major reason for the increase in the cost of care as doctors appear to frequently overprescribe tests or underutilize riskier, but more beneficial, treatment options as a matter of defensive medicine to protect themselves against threat of lawsuits (Sekhar and Vyas 2013).

As for the administrative issues associated with having seven different systems, this is a big problem. From the standpoint of economics, these administrative costs are basically transaction costs that serve as a tax on the provision of healthcare for everyone. If we look at the theory of the firm, we see that firms are, in fact, organized as a command-and-control system that then happen to operate within a free market. Why is it that we don't have everything covered by the free market and why do we use firms? Coase (1937) provides an answer for us – we use firms whenever the transaction costs of the market exceed the transaction costs of the firm. Currently, administrative costs for healthcare constitute more than a third of all costs for healthcare, while in Canada, which employs a single-payer system, administrative costs are only a sixth of all costs in healthcare (Himmelstein, Campbell, and Woolhandler 2020). This difference is even more meaningful when we consider that Canada spends considerably less than we do on healthcare.

The key issue is that these transaction costs will differ depending on the type of care. There are high transaction costs that accrue when one is attempting to determine who is a willing buyer and seller with emergency room care, especially since the person being cared for may not even be conscious at the time. Similarly, one has few options when it comes to ambulance service other than attempting to make Uber your ambulance service, which really only works when lifesaving equipment and medical staff are not immediately required such as is often the case with broken bones (Frankt 2018). This is a key reason why treating the emergency room in the same fashion as we do the police. On the other hand, primary care is probably something that can be done out of pocket for many individuals and if they were to face the cost after a certain number of covered visits, they would be less likely to call the doctor for minor ailments that they can treat themselves. Surgery and specialist care should probably be subject to outcomes-based payment structures and we should compensate primary care physicians who successfully treat patients by keeping them out of more expensive setting more as a reward for good work in order to shift the balance of care back to primary care and away from specialty care, which tends to be more expensive and less holistic in its approach.

We might consider whether our entire system needs to be overhauled. Currently we have a system that is based on sick care as opposed to healthcare. Our current system is reactive and based on treatment of sickness. There is little incentive to keep people well because doctors are primarily paid when we are sick. Thus we focus on treating symptoms rather than correcting underlying causes. We emphasize chronic care medications and treatments that keep us functional but fail to eliminate the actual problems. In many cases, healthcare providers actually propose interventions that are high-risk when there are other options still available. It is estimated that some 30% of all procedures in Canada are unnecessary and that is from a country that has a single-payer system (Canadian Institute for Health Information 2017). When you pay doctors on the basis of services performed, even if these services lead to good outcomes, you are still not incentivizing doctors to keep people well. Müllenbeck (2018) proposes that we no longer pay doctors on the basis of surgeries performed but rather on the basis of keeping patients well. This would move us to a capitation model in which insurance companies are paid a flat fee per subscriber but are completely responsible for medical care provision when the patients are sick. Similarly, all doctors and hospitals would be paid a single fee per day on the same basis. To ensure that patients do not engage in moral hazard, customers of these insurance companies would be required to "share their health data on a constant basis [including physical exams], monitoring of lifetime health data as well as genetic sequencing, cardiometabolic profiling and imaging-based technologies [...] to diminish their unique probability to fall sick of an identified, individual high-risk disease" (Müllenbeck 2018).

We also might want to consider whether we should be providing health insurance or prepaid medical care. Right now what we have is a system of prepaid medical care, not health insurance. If this were truly health insurance in the insurance sense of the term, many things that are currently covered would not be covered. Insurance is supposed to be used for unexpected severe expenses, which means that expenses that are neither unexpected nor severe should not be covered. By using insurance to pay for such things, we drive up the price of healthcare dramatically. We must remember that over 1/3 of *all* healthcare costs are administrative in nature, so if we can simplify the payment process, we can save hundreds of billions of dollars, lower premiums (or taxes if we wish to go to a single-payer plan), increase responsiveness of healthcare professionals, and guarantee price transparency since all costs are paid for in full and up front. It is true that this would mean greater out of pocket expenses at the healthcare provider but the overall cost to the consumer would be dramatically lower since premiums or taxes would be slashed. For individuals who are too poor to be able to afford these reduced costs, direct government subsidies, not unlike food stamps or housing assistance, can be provided.

A properly designed healthcare insurance program would cover major medical and emergency care only. Primary care doctors visits would be paid for completely out of pocket. This will stop people from running to the primary care doctor for simple things that can easily be cared for with over the counter medicines but will not prevent them from seeking out care for slightly more serious ailments. Expenses that are knowable or should be knowable in advance would not be covered. Thus, a normal pregnancy would not be covered but unexpected complications would definitely be covered. Co-insurance could be eliminated in favor of simply a deductible as is found in many other insurance plans. In cases of severe disease that ought to have been prevented, such as lung cancer for smokers or liver cancer for alcoholics, a decision could be made to not cover this expense, thus forcing people to engage in choices that are more responsible. Similarly, the obese could be denied treatment for certain diseases that are known to be highly correlated with obesity. If we do decide to go this route, a transition period would appear to be necessary and proper. Individuals who currently are smokers or alcoholics or overweight/obese would be grandfathered in provided they are making attempts to reduce or eliminate consumption of cigarettes, alcohol, or the excessive consumption of food. Still, we can imagine that such an imposition might be seen as overly strict despite the fact that it is common to use such criteria in the pricing of life insurance policies. If we fail to address behavioral habits that lead to poor health outcomes, we should expect that health insurance costs will be higher than necessary, but such a system may be necessary to make it palatable. After all, with 70.2% of all adults in the United States being overweight and 42.4% being obese, including obesity in the list of risks for which health coverage can be denied will likely be considered to be a very cruel way to allocate scarce health resources (Centers for Disease Control and Prevention 2021). This is especially true since obesity and poor eating habits often begin in childhood and to hold someone responsible for learned childhood behavior, even if it is known to be harmful, is not considering the fact the child did not have the mental or emotional competency to deviate from their parental instruction. Yet a similar argument surely needs to also be made for alcoholics since alcohol can be highly addictive and a good case may be made for drinking in moderation. Finally, smokers should also probably be exempted to nicotine's highly addictive nature, especially since smokers already contribute massive amounts of revenue to state and federal health agencies through cigarette taxation, effectively meaning that we have an unspoken social contract to take care of the consequences of their addiction. In other words, it is probably not something that we can do much about in this regard.

We should eliminate all certificate of need categories in their entirety. While it is perhaps legitimate to continue to require licensure to ensure quality of treatment, the certificate of need is simply a mechanism restricting an individual's or a company's ability to conduct business generally, which is fundamentally incompatible with any conception of fairness or free competition.

Sad as it is to say, we probably also are going to have to do something about the highly personalized medicine that is threatening to create a bifurcated society composed of those who can afford such treatments and those who cannot. If people can breed out of themselves and their genetic lines ailments but this selective use of genetics to create "designer babies" is not available to all, we may end up introducing particularly insidious forms of genetic determinism, scientific racism, and rampant discrimination under the guise of personal freedom (Comfort 2018). What exactly to do about this is difficult to say but in a country that already allow individuals to transfer much of their wealth to the succeeding generation, thus creating a vicious cycle that fosters intergeneration wealth inequality, the issue deserve serious attention. At some point, we need to realize that as inequality in all of its aspects increases, calls for reform will only grow stronger. Taking some steps to mitigate these inequities will ultimately create a more stable society than allowing them to grow unchecked. At the same time, restricting freedom too much will fundamentally alter the very nature of the country. What to do is not really an economics question. While economics can help us determine what is the punitive value of a statistical life, it cannot really assess what is the actual value to the individual of their own life or their lives of their children. However, anyone who argues that life is so priceless that it should not have a price needs to realize that we live in a world in which there is both limited and unequally allocated resources. The real question ends up being: how should we ultimately deal with the scarcity problem? Should we ration via the price system, allowing the richest among us to have the best care and denying to the poorest the same level because they are unable to afford it due to income or wealth constraints? Should we ration according to some third party, such as an insurance company or a government that uses a statistical value of life to assess how much your life is worth and whether it is worth saving denying to you agency over your own self? Should we ration as many countries do now by trying to thread the needle and provide a certain basic level of care for all but reserve the best care for those who can afford it, even if they have to travel outside of their own countries to get it, realizing it is impossible for all to have the best care given our limited resources. Ultimately, this is what economics really tells us: we cannot have what we want, everyone getting the very best standard of care available regardless of ability to pay, so we must settle on some second-best solution but what that will be is impossible for economics to give a definitive answer.

CONCLUSION

Economics can provide many insights into what is right and what is wrong with our current healthcare system but perhaps the most important insight is that it demonstrates that the current debate between Medicare-for-All versus our current system may be largely missing the point. We need to reduce the number of different systems operating in this country and the one chosen is less important than actually choosing just one. It is much less about who pays and much more about for what and why we pay that is key to cost-cutting in a manner that will prove beneficial to everyone. We need to look at our laws that create inefficiency and the administrative costs that reduce doctor and patient autonomy. Finally, we need to remember that economics cannot solve all of our issues; sometimes it can only illuminate our problems.

REFERENCES

Bank of America (2020). *2020 Workplace Benefits Report.*

Barone, E. (2020). How the New COVID-19 Pandemic Relief Bill Stacks Up to Other Countries' Economic Responses. *Time* https://time.com/5923840/us-pandemic-relief-bill-december/.

Beaton, T. (2017). What are the Pros and Cons of Consumer Directed Health Plans? *Health Pay Intelligence.* https://healthpayerintelligence.com/news/what-are-the-pros-and-cons-of-consumer-directed-health-plans.

Brownell, M. (2011). The WebMD Effect: Most Americans Are 'Cyberchondriacs. *The Street.* https://www.thestreet.com/personal-finance/insurance/webmd-effect-most-americans-are-cyberchondriacs-12789860.

Buchmueller, T. C., & Monheit, A. C. (2009). Employer-Sponsored Health Insurance and the Promise of Health Insurance Reform. *The Journal of Healthcare Organization, Provision, and Financing*, *46*(2), 187–202. doi:10.5034/inquiryjrnl_46.02.187 PMID:19694392

Bundorf, M. K. (2016). Consumer-Directed Health Plans: A Review of the Evidence. *The Journal of Risk and Insurance*, *83*(1), 9–41. doi:10.1111/jori.12141

C. I. A. (2021). *The World Factbook.* CIA. https://www.cia.gov/the-world-factbook/countries/

Centers for Disease Control and Prevention. (2021). Adult Obesity Facts. *CDC.* https://www.cdc.gov/obesity/data/adult.html.

Choosing Wisely Canada. (2017). *Unnecessary Care in Canada*. Canadian Institute for Health Information.

Chung, M. (2017). Healthcare Reform: Learning from Other Major Healthcare Systems. *Princeton Public Health Review*. https://pphr.princeton.edu/2017/12/02/unhealthy-health-care-a-cursory-overview-of-major-health-care-systems/.

Coase, R. (1937). The Nature of the Firm. *Economica*, *4*(16), 386–405. doi:10.1111/j.1468-0335.1937.tb00002.x

Cohen, R. A., Cha, A. E., Martinez, M. E., & Terlizzi, E. P. (2020). *Health Insurance Coverage: Early Release of Estimates From the National Health Interview Survey, 2019*. National Center for Health Statistics.

Comfort, N. (2018). Opening the Door to Eugenics. *MIT's Technology Review*, *121*(6), 16–19.

Cutler, D. M. (2004). *Your Money or Your Life: Strong Medicine for America's Healthcare System*. Oxford University Press.

DeVol, R. C., Bedroussian, A., & Yeo, B. (2011). *The Global Biomedical Industry: Preserving U.S. Leadership*. Milken Institute.

Ebhomielen, D. (2018). National Health Service England: An Overview and Analysis of Challenges. *Perspectives on Business and Economics*, *36*, 85–93.

Farrington, R. (2019). The Moral Hazard of Student Loan Forgiveness. *Forbes*. https://www.forbes.com/sites/robertfarrington/2019/06/25/the-moral-hazard-of-student-loan-forgiveness/?sh=56146b1e364c.

Fox, M. (2017). FDA Approves Pill That Tracks Whether You Took Your Meds. *NBC News*. http://nbcnews.com/health/health-news/fda-approves-pill-tracks-whether-you-took-your-meds-n820601, .

Frankt, A. (2018). Uber, Lyft and the Urgency of Saving Money on Ambulances. *The New York Times*, https://nytimes.com/2018/10/01/uber-lyft-and-the-urgency-of-saving-money-on-ambulances.html/.

Friedman, D. (2000). *Law's Order: What Economics Has to Do with Law and Why It Matters*. Princeton University Press.

Grossman, M. (1972a). *The Demand for Health: A Theoretical and empirical Investigation*. National Bureau of Economic Research.

Grossman, M. (1972b). On the Concept of Health Capital and the Demand for Health. *Journal of Political Economy*, *80*(March-April), 223–255. doi:10.1086/259880

Haviland, A. M., Eisenberg, M. D., Mehrotra, A., Huckfeldt, P. J., & Sood, N. (2016). Do 'Consumer-Directed' Health Plans Bend the Cost Curve Over Time? *Journal of Health Economics*, *46*(March), 33–51. doi:10.1016/j.jhealeco.2016.01.001 PMID:26851386

Heilbrun, J. (2013). Baumol's Cost Disease. In R. Towse (Ed.), *A Handbook of Cultural Economics* (pp. 67–75). Edward Elgar.

Helland, E., & Taborrok, A. (2019). *Why are the Prices So Damn High? Health, Education, and the Baumol Effect*. Mercatus Center, George Mason University.

Hercher, L. (2018). Are We Designing Inequality Into Our Genes? *MIT's Technology Review*, *121*(6), 68–69.

Hero, J. O., Zaslavsky, A. M., & Blendon, R. J. (2017). The United States Leads Other Nations in Differences by Income in Perceptions of Health and Healthcare. *Health Affairs*, *36*(6), 1032–1040. doi:10.1377/hlthaff.2017.0006 PMID:28583961

Hicks, L. L. (2021). *Economics of Health and Medical Care*. Jones and Bartlett Learning.

Himmelstein, D. U., Campbell, T., & Woolhandler, S. (2020). Heath Care Administrative Costs in the United States and Canada, 2017. *Annals of Internal Medicine*, *172*(2), 134–142. doi:10.7326/M19-2818 PMID:31905376

Hoffower, H. (2020). More than a quarter of indebted millennials said they didn't know what they were signing up for with their student loans. *Business Insider.* https://www.businessinsider.com/millennials-dont-understand-student-loan-terms-interest-2020-1.

Koopman, C., & Stratmann, T. (2015). *Certificate of Need Laws: Implications for North Carolina*. Mercatus Institute, George Mason University.

Luft, H. S. (2006). What Works and What Doesn't Work Well in the US Healthcare System. *PharmacoEconomics*, *24*(S2), 15–28. doi:10.2165/00019053-200624002-00003 PMID:23389485

Luxottica (2021). Homepage. *Luxottica.* https://www.luxottica.com/en/.

Madjd-Sadjadi, Z. (2016). *The Economics of Civil and Common Law*. Business Expert Press.

Mannion, R., & Davies, H. T. O. (2008). Payment for performance in health care. *BMJ (Clinical Research Ed.)*, *336*(7639), 306–308. doi:10.1136/bmj.39463.454815.94 PMID:18258966

Martin, A. B., Hartman, M., Lassman, D., & Catlin, A. (2020). National Healthcare Spending in 2019: Steady Growth for the Fourth Consecutive Year. *Health Affairs*, *40*(1), 14–24. doi:10.1377/hlthaff.2020.02022 PMID:33326300

Mcaskill, R. (2014). Examining Differences Between Medicare, Medicaid Reimbursement. *Revcycle Intelligence*. https://revcycleintelligence.com/news/examining-differences-medicare-medicaid-reimbursement.

McDonald, R., S. Harrison, K. Checkland, S. M. Campbell, and M. Roland (2007). Impact of Financial Incentives on Clincial Autonomy and Internal Motivation in Primary Care: Ethnographic Study. *BMJ*, . doi:10.1136/bmj.39238.890810.BE

Müllenbeck, M. (2018). What if we Paid Doctors to Keep People Healthy? *TED Talks*. https://www.ted.com/talks/matthias_mullenbeck_what_if_we_paid_doctors_to_keep_people_healthy/transcript?language=en, accessed on April 7, 2021.

Observatory of Economic Complexity. (2021). *Medical Instruments*. https://oec.world/en/profile/hs92/medical-instruments

OECD. (2021). *OECD Statistics*. [Data set]. http://stats.oecd.org.

Penn, M., Bhatnagar, S., Kuy, S., Liberman, S., Elnahal, S., Clancy, C., & Shulkin, D. (2019). Comparison of Wait Times for New Patients Between the Private Sctor and the United States Department of Veterans Affairs Medical Centers. *JAMA Network Open*, *2*(1), e187096. doi:10.1001/jamanetworkopen.2018.7096 PMID:30657532

Pione, A. (2018). One Tumor at a Time. *MIT's Technology Review*, *121*(6), 46–51.

Reed, R. O. B. R., & Sood, N. (2017). Impact of Consumer-Directed Health Plans on Low-Value Healthcare. *The American Journal of Managed Care*, *23*(12), 741–748. PMID:29261240

Regalado, A. (2018). A Cure for One. *MIT's Technology Review*, *121*(6), 38–45.

Richardson, C., Hall, M., & Madjd-Sadjadi, Z. (2010). Lessons from Credit Bureaus for Improving the Market for Electronic Medical Records. *The Journal of Consumer Affairs*, *44*(3), 546–556. doi:10.1111/j.1745-6606.2010.01183.x

Sekhar, M. S., & Vyas, N. (2013). Defensive Medicine: A Bane to Healthcare. *Annals of Medical and Health Sciences Research*, *3*(2), 295–296. doi:10.4103/2141-9248.113688 PMID:23919211

Smith, P. C. (1995). On the Unintended Consequences of Publishing Performance Data in the Public Sector. *International Journal of Public Administration*, *18*(2-3), 277–310. doi:10.1080/01900699508525011

Spitzer, J. (2018). Medical Record Errors are Common, Hard to Fix, Report Says. *Beckers Hospital Review*. https://www.beckershospitalreview.com/ehrs/medical-record-errors-are-common-hard-to-fix-report-finds.html.

Statista. (2021). Coronavirus (COVID-19) deaths worldwide per one million population as of March 5, 2021, by country. *Statista*. https://www.statista.com/statistics/1104709/coronavirus-deaths-worldwide-per-million-inhabitants/ .

Thompson, D. (2021). US Life Expectancy Drops 1 Full Year Due to COVID-19. *WebMD*. https://www.webmd.com/lung/news/20210218/us-life-expectancy-drops-1-full-year-due-to-covid19#1.

Weil, T. P. (2016). What can the Canadians and Americans learn from each other's healthcare systems? *The International Journal of Health Planning and Management*, *31*(3), 349–370. doi:10.1002/hpm.2374 PMID:27469581

Wenz, P. S. (2015). *Functional Inefficiency: The Unexpected Benefits of Wasting Time and Money*. Prometheus Books.

Wolf, C. Jr. (1988). *Markets or Governments: Choosing Between Imperfect Alternatives*. MIT Press.

World Health Organization. (1946). Preamble to the Constitution of WHO as adopted by the International Health Conference (Official Records of WHO, no. 2, p. 100).

World Health Organization. (2021a). *Global Health Expenditure Database*. [Data set]. https://apps.who.int/nha/database/Select/Indicators/en.

World Health Organization. (2021b). *Global Health Observatory Data Repository*. [Data set]. https://apps.who.int/gho/data/view.main.SDG2016LEXv?lang=en.

Yee, T., A. E. Lechner, and E. R. Boukus (2013). *The Surge in Urgent Care Centers: Emergency Department Alternative or Costly Convenience, Research Brief 26*. Center for Studying Health System Change .

Zhang, X., Trish, E., & Sood, N. (2018). Financial Burden of Healthcare Utilization in Consumer-Directed Health Plans. *The American Journal of Managed Care*, *24*(4), e115–e121. PMID:29668214

Section 2

Technological and Human Capital Challenges

Chapter 5
Effective Technological Progress as a Contributing Factor to an Improved Health System in the United States

Nikolaos Karagiannis
Winston-Salem State University, USA

Aparna A. Gosavi
Winston-Salem State University, USA

Abhijit Gosavi
Missouri University of Science and Technology, USA

ABSTRACT

The U.S. government and its population incurs more out-of-pocket expenses in terms of per capita than ever before. The question that arises as a result is: does the increased expenditure result in either improved quality or quicker access to healthcare? To answer this question, the role modern technology plays in the deliverance of healthcare is analyzed in this chapter. An important conclusion that can be drawn from this analysis is that the U.S. needs to fund research to develop, monitor, and implement healthcare technologies that will allow physicians to supplement and improve their practices. Further, capacity management of beds and increased investment into healthcare in general appears to be critical, regardless of how effectively technology is used.

DOI: 10.4018/978-1-6684-4060-5.ch005

INTRODUCTION

Healthcare costs –government and out-of-pocket– in the U.S. are on the rise. For example, from 2011 to 2018, the increase in the US government healthcare expenditure (per capita) was 35.52 percent while the same number for the European Union was 0.77 percent (Figure 1).

Figure 1. Government healthcare expenditure per capita, current US$
Source: The World Development Indicators, 2021[1]

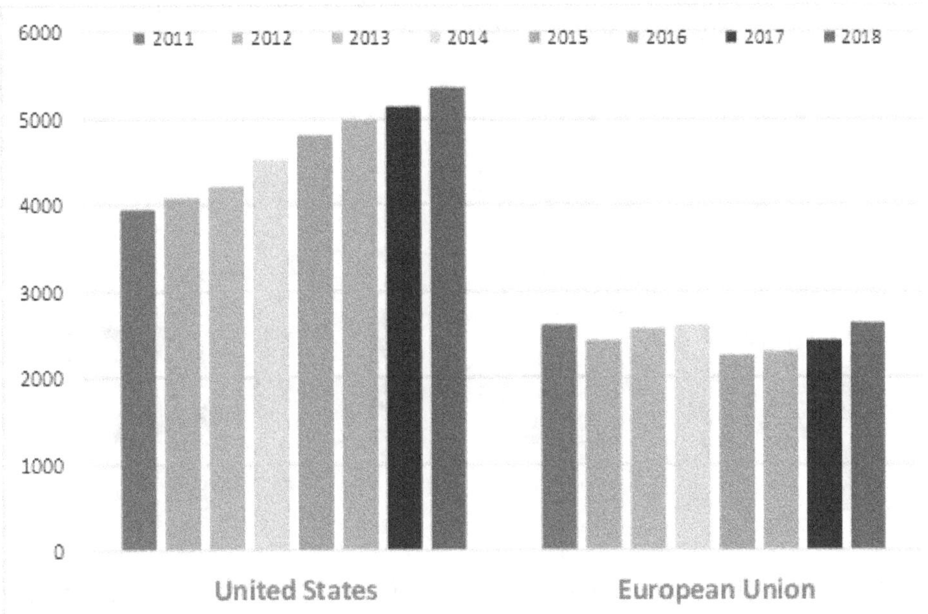

The US population experienced a 15.26 percent *increase* in out-of-pocket expenditures (Figure 2), whereas people across the Atlantic enjoyed a 3 percent *decrease*. These numbers certainly demand analysis. When our government in terms of per capita and the population in terms of out-of-pocket pay more dollars for healthcare than ever before, the obvious question is: does it result in improved quality or quicker access to healthcare? To answer this question, we look at the role modern technology plays in the deliverance of healthcare.

Despite expectations to the contrary, challenges in delivering high-quality healthcare appear to be intensifying in many of the world's most developed countries, including in the United States, during an era of rapid innovative technological developments and global pandemics. Technological developments are expected to impact the quality of healthcare, although change has been reported to be difficult to implement.[2] These technological developments have been better adopted and utilized in healthcare fields in some parts of the world than in others. In general, developed nations have been able to harness technology more efficiently for improved patient care (Heathcare Tech Outlook, 2020).[3] As the quantification of health in modern society intensifies and innovative health technologies become the cornerstone of these developments, the connection between technology and healthcare is garnering increased attention.

Figure 2. Out-of-pocket healthcare expenditure per capita, current US$
Source: The World Development Indicators, 2021

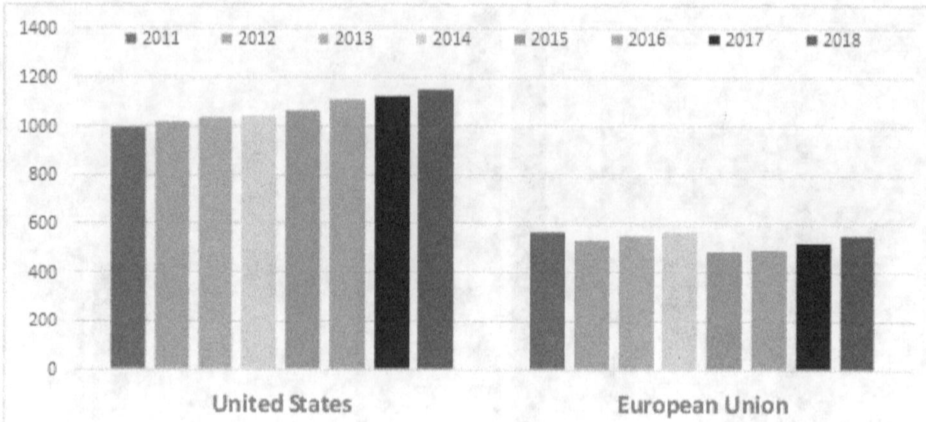

Recent years have witnessed an era of intensified technology use in healthcare services as well as developments in personalized medicine. These advances have promoted a growing dependency on technology in society and the collection of advanced information, which are then used to influence the decisions and behaviors of not just ordinary citizens but also large institutions, health personnel, and private companies.

Healthcare technology refers to information technology (IT) tools or software designed to boost hospital and administrative efficiency and productivity, give new insights into medicines and treatments, or improve the overall quality of care provided. Several innovations are generally seen as positive developments, improving the diagnostics and treatment of diseases as well as general public health; however, their wider societal implications can be questioned. It appears likely that these technologies could be improving general public health but at the cost of overall coverage and greater efficiency in healthcare provision. The U.S. healthcare system is not well designed to provide *equitable* care, as evidenced by the prevalence of disparities in care by race, ethnicity, language, and social status. As the United States invests in the design and implementation of health IT, consideration must be given to the impact that these innovations have on the quality and cost of healthcare for all patients, including those who experience difficulties.

Racial and ethnic disparities in healthcare have been consistently documented in the diagnosis, treatment, and outcomes of many common clinical conditions as new medical technologies and innovativeness have been used at different rates among different ethnic groups. These differences in innovativeness are associated with significant racial differences in response to particular healthcare technologies. Healthcare providers who haven't yet adopted the tools technology places at their disposal are realizing their vast untapped potential and are making the changes and the investments required to streamline processes, lower costs, increase efficiency and, most importantly, to improve quality of care. Development of an IT infrastructure should address disparities in care from the start. Information technology alone cannot eliminate disparities, but as we harness its full potential to improve quality, we should ensure that disparities are not simply an afterthought for IT. Only a thoughtfully designed and implemented IT system will be capable of improving the general health quality– and in the process address disparities in healthcare.

Moreover, it is not sufficient to focus attention solely on healthcare services technologies, but investigating emerging technologies in lifestyle health, genomics, and the increased use of personalized devices in health is equally critical. A deeper understanding of social inequalities in health and innovative health technologies is dependent on distinguishing between a perspective focused on individual resource use, technology access/use, and health outcomes, and a perspective focused on mechanisms that are more dependent on social and institutional structure than on individual agency. However, it is becoming increasingly important to investigate main implications and consequences of a society increasingly influenced by technological innovations, including the ways in which these technologies may influence the unequal distribution of health.

The focus of this chapter is to provide a better understanding of the complex relationships between innovative health technologies and greater overall efficiency. Factors and mechanisms that influence access, for example, may differ from factors and mechanisms that influence use. It is clear that it is not enough to solely focus on factors and mechanisms that influence unequal access and, therefore, ignore how variations in use importantly shape inequalities and inefficiencies in health. The chapter also suggests that a public policy perspective can benefit from a better understanding, and differentiation, of technologies based on how these technologies are accessed and used by end users.

The Diffusion of Modern Technology: Costs and Benefits to Healthcare

Technologies are praised for saving lives, improving health status, and improving the quality of care. Ideally, technology can facilitate providers' ability to offer care to more people. At the same time, modern technology is often criticized as one dominant factor responsible for the continuing escalation of medical costs. Highly important treatments, such as diagnostic imaging systems, new biotechnology products and organ transplantation, attract both approval and responsibility. Healthcare changes dramatically because of technological developments, from anesthetics and antibiotics to magnetic resonance imaging scanners and radiotherapy. Future technological innovation is likely to keep transforming healthcare, yet, while technologies (new drugs and treatments, new devices, new social media support for healthcare, etc.) will drive innovation, human factors will remain one of the stable limitations of breakthroughs.

Several factors related to new medical technologies are considered in this chapter. First, modern technologies improve the quality of medical care by improving health outcomes. This is not true of every technology in every clinical use, but is true in general. Second, many new technologies are ineffective or redundant and do not improve health outcomes. The challenge is that it is not always easy to discriminate between effective and ineffective technologies at the time they are introduced. Third, new technologies add to healthcare costs. Some technologies may actually reduce costs by replacing more expensive alternatives or preventing expensive health consequences, but the overall effect is to increase costs. Fourth, the incentives and regulations built into the American healthcare sector lead to inappropriate diffusion of technologies, both under-diffusion of effective technologies and over-diffusion of ineffective technologies. Professional reward structures, compensation systems, legal and ethical considerations, and patient demands all contribute to the problem. The fifth fact about new medical technology is that the American public cannot get enough of it since Americans demand the best and newest from the healthcare providers.

Upward pressures on healthcare costs have been increasing since the 1990s (Figures 1 and 2). A growing array of technological advances claim an increasingly large share of national resources. What is concerning is that out-of-pocket expenses for the population have increased (Figure 2), while the capacity of beds has decreased significantly on a per capita basis (Figure 3). The total impact of a technology on healthcare costs is broad and may include offsetting savings as well as induced costs. Medical technologies, especially new ones, will have to justify their costs in a climate of competing claims on resources. Researchers generally agree that medical technology has contributed to rising healthcare costs. Some researchers have even tried to estimate the effect of technology on U.S. healthcare expenditures by estimating the impact of other, more easily identifiable sources including increase in prices and age-specific population growth. The portion of the increase in health spending not accounted for by these explanatory variables is attributed to technology.

Figure 3. Hospital beds per 1000 (Source: The World Development Indicators, 2021)
Source: The World Development Indicators, 2021

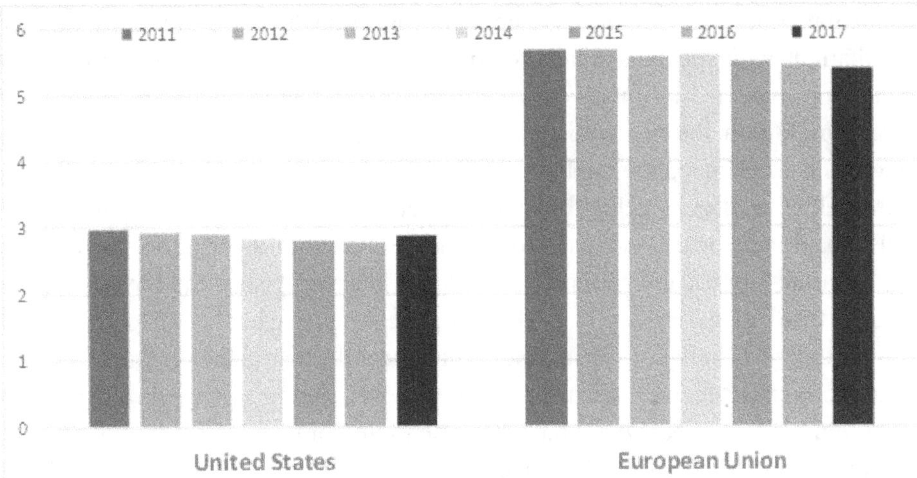

The consequences of technological advancement for work and workers depends on how it is put to use towards addressing the shared objectives guiding the healthcare industry. Yet, researchers have struggled to measure how much technology has contributed to increasing costs. Such research does not distinguish between expanded applications of existing technologies and introduction of new technologies. Even if the more important innovations are taken into account, it would be very difficult to trace their overall economic impact. In addition, these studies do not easily identify indirect costs of using new technologies, such as, the need for more skilled healthcare professionals and technicians, nor do they identify induced costs. These limitations may force institutionalized interventions, challenging the fallacy of "best available technology for all."

The problem is that costs continue to rise, and the ability of the public and private sectors to finance healthcare is being strained. American society may have reached the point at which it is not possible to provide the best available healthcare to every American, regardless of cost. The direct effect has been to restrict access to healthcare for a growing segment of the population –the uninsured– while preserving the illusion of best available care for those fortunate enough to have coverage. Health insurance can remove financial barriers to consumers, thus, raising demand for technology and inducing providers to offer a more affordable mix of services. Universal health insurance may well be adopted. The main criterion should be based on the proposition that the objective of medical technology is to improve health outcomes.

Unprecedented challenges confront the U.S. healthcare sector. Technology has brought about a massive and welcome change to the healthcare industry. Patients now have access to some of the best diagnostic tools, new and cutting-edge treatments, and many minimally invasive procedures resulting in less pain and quicker recovery. Telemedicine facilitates remote patient monitoring by healthcare professions. Remote consultations with specialists, targeted treatments, and the availability of intuitive mobile apps have led to improved patient care and a better healthcare experience overall. In addition, the availability of newer treatment technologies leading to better outcomes has enhanced the quality of life of the patients as well.

In healthcare, digital technology and artificial intelligence could help transform unsustainable healthcare systems into sustainable ones, align the relationship between medical professionals and patients, and provide cheaper, faster, and more effective solutions for diseases. Evidently, the U.S. healthcare system has begun to implement some noteworthy changes to its infrastructure under the continued pressure from the pandemic. Various technological solutions that were being slowly introduced into the system before the pandemic have become more dominant nowadays. One such solution, telemedicine, is used in diverse sectors including cardiology, radiology, behavioral health, and others. Even after the pandemic subsides, many patients and other potential customers may prefer a virtual consultation option,[4] as it reduces the cost of healthcare related services such as hospital stays and is also safer. This shift, in turn, could help provide momentum to new healthcare models in telemedicine.

Current global pandemics, such as the spread of COVID-19, have exposed and amplified many of the underlying weaknesses of the U.S. system, including a lack of widespread access to care, inefficiencies, and runaway costs. The U.S. healthcare industry also lags behind other domestic industries and other countries' healthcare systems in terms of technology adoption. COVID-19 may speed up technological changes like the use of telemedicine. These technological changes are also expected to further transform service delivery and scale up the utilization of digital systems as digital transformation could make the difference in delivery and cost. Besides, the health industry's desire for data has grown beyond medical histories. To provide better and cheaper services, healthcare professionals are now collecting specialized information and data.

There seems to be an untapped potential for new technology to propel changes in healthcare delivery. This untapped potential is centered around two significant research questions: 1. What are the new technologies that have the potential to affect employment, wages, skill requirements, and work organization? And 2. What are the potential consequences of these technologies for different healthcare occupations, and how are those effects likely to vary by race, ethnicity, gender, age, and educational attainment? While some new technologies may be able to improve outcomes both for patients and for healthcare providers, this is not a foregone conclusion. The consequences of technological change in healthcare will ultimately depend on the choices policy-makers and industry stakeholders make in this current time of crisis and in the future.

OTHER RELATED CHALLENGES

While forms of technology in healthcare may have made positive changes in the world, there is evidence for the negative physical health and psychological effects of modern technology and its overuse in addition to unsolved problems in medicine. Privacy, disinformation, cyberattacks, cloud computing, automation, and ethics challenges for artificial intelligence are (should be) vital priorities that modern technology needs to continually be addressing and can do more to help advance. During the last three years or so, privacy protection has spread and deepened in the United States and most countries of the world. The facial recognition issues took center stage, driven in part by concerns by academics and civil liberties groups about risks of discrimination and the potential impact on privacy and other democratic rights. As digital becomes the default, institutions must be extra vigilant in the detection and prevention of cyber threats.

Perhaps the most fundamental and direct impact that new technology has on the everyday life of most people is economic in nature. The issue of jobs and unemployment is one that raises serious concerns in many people. While competition between machinery and human labor has long existed in the realm of physical tasks, it has only recently been introduced into the domain of mental work. Much as heavy machinery has eliminated the need for physical exertion on the part of humans, so too does modern technology, in the form of microchips and computers, for example. Moreover, during the same period, the public's anxiety over the impact of artificial intelligence on the economy and jobs continued to grow. Especially in the United States and Europe, people questioned whether modern technology will destroy more jobs than it will create. However, there also emerged a new recognition that continuing prosperity will require productivity advances from technology to offer new solutions to societal problems, with immigration and diversity remaining front and center.

Redefining necessary healthcare skills has been a complicated challenge as educational initiatives, technological advances, societal dynamics, and the empowerment of students and young adults affect the presence of essential skills in the healthcare sector. Besides, the "digital divide" mirrors recent increases in technology use by racial and ethnic minorities. Consequently, there can be an overall mismatch between technological advancement and existing skills. Such a gap in skills exists because the American society has evolved. Just as technology and medicine can provide advances and life-sustaining products, people must also evolve to foster a better human capital connection.

In the United States and several other countries, the last three years brought a continuing focus on challenges for rural communities too. Leveraging computers and mobile devices to understand one's health, support self-management, and interact with providers is associated with favorable health outcomes. However, not everyone uses these technologies, potentially limiting broad benefits, especially in rural communities. Increased reliance on technology to promote patient health may have limited value if certain geographical areas and groups lack access and/or the skills to leverage these tools. Often times, what's good for high technology companies may challenge a community as there may be limited benefits and externalities from direct investments in high technology sectors (including healthcare). Technology is going to change and shape the medical industry for decades to come. Implementing technology in medicine has also a steep learning curve. Those who need this new technology most may not have time to learn how to use it. But without a comprehensive understanding, trying to use medical technology can lead to practitioner error and malpractice. Hospital administrators, medical professionals and IT teams need to tackle this challenge head-on. Those that don't adapt will be left behind, struggling to keep up with the wave of innovation that's sweeping through healthcare.

THE WAY FORWARD

Given the challenges facing the healthcare industry in the United States and the opportunities that new technologies present, the choices we make now can lead us in one of two directions. Policy makers and industry leaders can choose a high-road path, in which the benefits of technological change are shared among patients, providers, and healthcare workers alike. Or, they can continue along the default trajectory, in which technology is deployed primarily to increase returns for atomized actors, and to reduce staffing and increase micromanagement of workers. Taking the high road will require coordinated efforts to improve industry outcomes that involve a voice for all stakeholders. The future of healthcare lies in working hand-in-hand with technology, and healthcare workers have to embrace emerging healthcare technologies in order to stay relevant in the coming years with a view that interventions, learning, adaptation, and experimentation may never end.

The U.S. healthcare sector has a history of underperformance in the areas of access, cost, and quality. The COVID-19 pandemic has further exposed the frailty and ineffectiveness of the system and pointed to the need to leverage technology towards a more efficient use of the healthcare workforce. Technology can play an important role in moving the nation toward the healthcare high road. New technologies must be evaluated as early as possible and should be reevaluated frequently. Both health and economic impact should be part of these evaluations. The role of information and guidelines for cost-effective care would be enhanced in such an environment, and the research base for providing such information in real time should be expanded. The voice of the American public cannot be ignored. The people want cost containment, but they also want new technology if it can bring them better healthcare. A system that rewards cost-effective healthcare and encourages cost-effective new technology could accomplish both objectives.

Public-private partnerships can expand important technological equipment, and can help with human resource training, retraining and retooling while promoting increased public access to vital health services. The unique manner in which the United States delivers, and finances healthcare seems to provide a guarantee that present market forces will not beget obstacles to leverage the use of new technologies for improvements in industry performance and worker well-being. Without careful, coordinated decision-making, technological choices are likely to undermine workers' job quality and their ability to exercise their voice at work. The effect of this will be to limit the possible ways in which technology could be used to improve outcomes for patients, providers, front-line workers, taxpayers, and society at large.

In order to achieve a better health system for all in the United States, the following related broad areas need to be emphasized:

- strengthening health information technology regulation.
- bridging the digital gap between healthcare organizations.
- providing better preventive services and safer healthcare.
- defining higher quality measures; and
- improving the accessibility of health information for patients.

Although there are several telehealth programs that cater to several rural communities, for instance, in the Midwest, there are ways to extend this coverage to rural areas in all 50 states. This solution should be developed in a way that uses already existing technologies as pilot models and is adapted to fit the needs of specific geographical regions. Partnering with regional and state medical boards will allow this process to be streamlined, while focusing on eliminating limitations.

Looking at all of these broad areas, policy should be developed in a way that allows a step-by-step rollout of healthcare technology as well as education and training programs. Overall, redefining the boundaries of healthcare technology policy and research with the support of health institutions, physicians, and other healthcare providers will allow for management of chronic and complex conditions and improve access to healthcare.

CONCLUSION

The implementation of healthcare technology in a variety of different medical settings will allow for a better healthcare system in the United States. From increasing federal funding for medical devices and telemedicine to the development of education and implementation programs, the United States needs to fund research to develop, monitor, and implement healthcare technology and generate healthcare policy that will benefit the citizens and allow physicians to supplement and improve their practices. Capacity management of beds and increased investment into healthcare in general appears to be critical regardless of how effectively technology is used.

REFERENCES

Braithwaite, J. (2018). Changing how we think about healthcare improvement. *BMJ (Clinical Research Ed.)*, *361*, k2014. doi:10.1136/bmj.k2014 PMID:29773537

Gilbert, A. W., Billany, J. C., Adam, R., Martin, L., Tobin, R., Bagdai, S., Galvin, N., Farr, I., Allain, A., Davies, L., & Bateson, J. (2020). Rapid implementation of virtual clinics due to COVID-19: Report and early evaluation of a quality improvement initiative. *BMJ Open Quality*, *9*(2), e000985. doi:10.1136/bmjoq-2020-000985 PMID:32439740

Heathcare Tech Outlook. (2020), How Technology is Helping HeathCare System to Improve Care. *Healthcare Tech.* https://www.healthcaretechoutlook.com/news/how-technology-is-helping-healthcare-system-to-improve-care-nid-1942.html

The World Bank. (2022). *Databank: World Development Indicators.* https://databank.worldbank.org/reports.aspx?source=World-Development-Indicators

Chapter 6
Telehealth and Telemedicine: Challenges and Prospects in Healthcare Delivery

Stephanie Joseph
Winston-Salem State University, USA

Benjamin Philip Greene
Independent Researcher, USA

ABSTRACT

This chapter examines the utilization of telehealth from its inception to the recent prodigious increase in utilization during the Covid-19 pandemic. Delivery methods, including synchronous and asynchronous methods as well as remote and mobile health, are described. Its history and utilization in rural and exceptional settings and its comparative efficacy with traditional care are reviewed. Legal questions, including those related to autonomy, confidentiality, licensing, and jurisdictional concerns are presented. Finally, trends and a review of the prospects for the future of telehealth are examined.

INTRODUCTION: WHAT IS TELEHEALTH?

The terms telehealth and telemedicine are used interchangeably by both medical personnel and the general public, however, there are differences between the two. In a Department of Health and Human Services (DHHS) posting, last reviewed on October 17, 2019, in HealthIT.gov, DHHS describes each: "Telehealth is different from telemedicine because it refers to a *broader scope of remote healthcare services* than telemedicine. While telemedicine refers specifically to remote clinical services,"

DOI: 10.4018/978-1-6684-4060-5.ch006

telehealth is more expansive including "non-clinical services, such as medical training, administrative meetings, and continuing medical education, in addition to clinical services" (The Office of the National Coordinator for Health Information Technology (ONC), 2019).

Telehealth delivery methods have been instrumental in tackling the disparity in quality of, and access to, care for those in remote areas. Four methods have proven especially effective:

1. *Synchronous Live Videoconferencing*: Connecting provider and patient for virtual appointments.
2. *Asynchronous Store-and-Forward*: The provider and patient do not meet in person or virtually. Instead, healthcare information is transmitted as a data package and stored for later review.
3. *Remote Patient Monitoring*: Technologies that allow the provider to monitor health from a distance, such as devices that measure, record, and wirelessly transmit data.
4. *Mobile Health*: Use of personal health apps on digital devices, such as smartphones and tablets, that can provide a patient the ability to calculate, record, and store personal health information (Mayo Clinic, 2020).

HISTORY OF TELEHEALTH IN THE U.S.

The history of Telehealth includes the historic first telephone call between Alexander Graham Bell and Thomas A. Watson when Bell said "Mr. Watson, come here; I want you." He was seeking medical assistance after spilling sulfuric acid on his pants on March 10, 1876 (Aronson, 1977). A few years later, a physician was called by a worried mother to ask if her child had croup. He asked to listen to the child's cough and assured the mother that it was not croup. This conversation was reported in an 1879 article in the medical journal, *Lancet* that discussed the telephone as a means to reduce unnecessary office visits (Board on Health Care Services; Institute of Medicine., 2012). Other early events include the delivery of medical services by radio to researchers in Antarctica in the early 1900s (Maheu, et al., 2002), and the publication of a paper on the telecardiogram by the inventor of the electrocardiogram in 1906. Figure 1 from the 1925 cover of *Science and Invention* magazine featured a doctor diagnosing a patient by radio, and contemplated the video examination in the same issue of *Science and Invention* of a patient over distance (Board on Health Care Services; Institute of Medicine., 2012) using a machine of the future called the Teledactyl (Novak, 2012). In the 1940s, radiology images were transmitted between two Pennsylvania towns in the first known example of a medical record

Figure 1. A physicin utilizing the "Teledactyl"

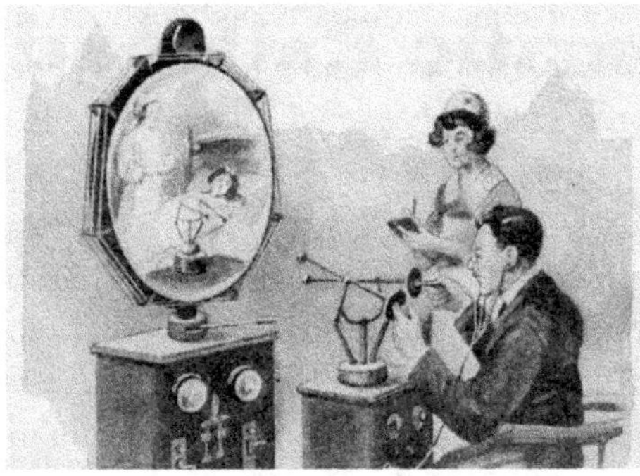

transfer (eVisit, 2021). Telepathology, telepharmacology, and teledentistry have all been used for years (Board on Health Care Services; Institute of Medicine., 2012).

Although telemedicine and telehealth have a long history, they have been primarily opportunistic in methodology and scope and were primarily utilized by government agencies where reimbursement was not an issue and patient-to-facility remoteness presented a challenge. As an example, the need for a unique way to treat astronauts participating in human spaceflight and International Space Station (ISS) missions prompted the development of a telemedicine application. This capability was tested when an astronaut aboard the ISS developed a deep vein thrombosis (DVT) in the jugular vein. Physicians and scientists at the National Aeronautics and Space Administration (NASA) worked with a doctor from the University of North Carolina (UNC) Blood Research Center to permit continuous health monitoring, ultrasound analyses of the clot, medication management and supply capabilities during resupply missions from the earth. As a result of this experience, the need for innovative methods to monitor the status of astronauts was identified (Wicklund, 2020). Interestingly, the blood clot was originally discovered by the astronaut when he underwent an ultrasound of his neck for a research study on how body fluid is redistributed in zero gravity (UNC School of Medicine, 2020).

Back on earth, the U.S. Department of Veterans Affairs (VA) has a long history of the utilization of telehealth and telemedicine. Their Office of Rural Health Programs operates teleintensive care units, telemental health hubs, veteran transportation services, remote telephone-based cardiac rehabilitation programs, and service to special populations, including Indian Health Services and Women Veterans programs (Office of the National Coordinator for Health Information Technology Federal Office of Rural Health Policy - Health Resources and Services Administration, 2016). As an example, the Cardiac Rehabilitation case management program begins with an in-person visit with a specialist to help the veteran safely learn rehabilitation exercises.

Subsequent sessions occur at home and are conducted using virtual interaction with rehabilitation staff. In this instance, comparisons between fully in-person and virtual programs indicated a comparable cost and a lack of negative impacts from remote care. Remote patients reported higher satisfaction levels and a greater likelihood to achieve program completion.

The Department of Defense (DOD) also utilizes telehealth to provide care to patients located throughout the world and is building both synchronous and asynchronous teleconsultation capability. In a review of its teledermatology program between 2004 and 2012, teleconsultation with the patient resulted in a reduction of 46 dermatologic evacuations from duty and the facilitation of 41 evacuations in a manner that permitted 98% of the consultations to occur within 24 hours and 23% within one hour (Capt. Jane S. Hwang & Charles M. Lappan, 2014). A similar result was noted in a 2020 journal article which concluded that the introduction of a Health Experts online Portal (HELP) might help to manage routine non-battle injury medical issues and reduce medical evacuations (MEDEVACs). In this study, the use of asynchronous telemedicine in Iraq and Syria resulted in a reduction of MEDEVACs from 157 to 68, or a 56.7% reduction

Figure 2. Federal agencies and their telehealth utilization
(Office of the National Coordinator for Health Information Technology, 2016)

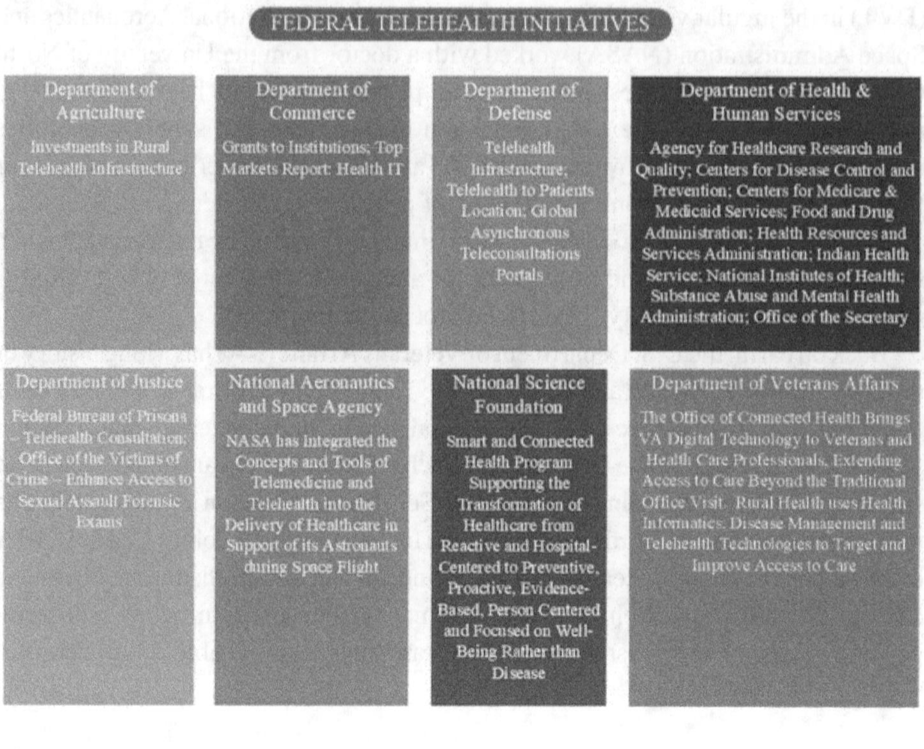

Figure 2 displays the utilization of telehealth by other federal agencies in a variety of fashions:

TELEHEALTH AND TELEMEDICINE IN RURAL AND EXCEPTIONAL SETTINGS

Rural communities often face multiple barriers to accessing healthcare. The CMS Rural Health Council (RH Council) was developed in 2016 to address these issues by providing recommendations for impactful policies and regulations. One of the RH Council's strategic initiatives includes providing tools for people in those populations to obtain better access to care and is focused on "ensuring access to high-quality health care to all Americans in rural settings (CMS.gov, 2020)."

Well in advance of the Rural Health Council, substantive utilization of rural telemedicine and telehealth in the United States occurred dating back to the 1970s under a public and private partnership involving NASA, the Papago Tribe of Southern Arizona (now the Tohono O'odham Indian Nation), General Electric, Boeing, the Lockheed Martin Missile and Space Company, the Indian Health Service and the Department of Health, Education and Welfare (HEW). Named the Space Technology Applied to Rural Papago Advanced Health Care (STARPAHC) project, this involved the utilization of remote healthcare space technology to serve remote populations on earth. Health disparities for Native peoples were significantly worse than the general population even with the founding of the Indian Health Service (IHS) in 1955 and efforts to expand medical facilities in the 1960s. Native peoples' life expectancy was nearly six years lower than the general population. Concurrently, the Nixon administration encouraged a more practical return on investment from NASA. Satellite experiments using the Applications Technology Satellite (ATS-1) to connect nine remote Alaskan villages with physicians improved the diagnosis of illness among the connected group more than in the control group of four villages that did not have satellite ground stations. Subsequent larger satellites allowed for the transmission of video through Health Education Technology (HET) experiments. The primary benefit of these collaborative efforts was to demonstrate the effectiveness of telemedicine for remote communities, a recognition of the potential benefit of telehealth during space exploration, and collaborative methods to achieve medical breakthroughs (Simpson, et al., 2020). Early efforts of this type most certainly influenced the later inclusion of telemedicine reimbursement for rural health by the Centers for Medicare and Medicaid Services (CMS) and the utilization of telehealth by the Department of Veterans Affairs.

Remote health solutions include the provision of medicine to drilling platforms located hundreds of miles offshore thereby permitting access to specialists and reducing travel-related costs. Home monitoring of patients with chronic conditions permits improved interaction with specialists and improved outcomes. In the case of diabetes, patients using both insulin pumps and continuous glucose monitors receive glucose level reports every five minutes and they can adjust the delivery of insulin or carbohydrates to address both high and low levels. Recent Pump software automatically delivers doses of insulin or stops deliveries of insulin and warns the user of undesirable trends. In addition, historical and real-time data is uploaded to physician offices for their review and assessment in advance of in-person office visits.

As of April of 2018, CMS began covering rural telehealth services under Part B via an interactive videoconference between a practitioner located at a distant site and a patient located at a certified rural originating site. Initially, the originating site was required to be an authorized medical facility and typically could not be a beneficiary's home or office. Additionally, distant site practitioners had to be licensed to provide services in the patient's state and could be either physicians, nurse practitioners, or physician assistants. There was standardized reimbursement when an interactive audio and video telecommunications system was used. Also, Medicare would pay for asynchronous store and forward technology when the originating site was part of a federal telemedicine demonstration project, in Alaska or Hawaii. Eligible originating sites are located in a county outside of a metropolitan statistical area (MSA); in a health professional shortage area (HPSA) or a site that is participating in a Federal telemedicine demonstration project approved by or funded by the Secretary of Health and Human Services (Department of Health and Human Services Office of Inspector General, 2018).

TELEHEALTH AND TELEMEDICINE IN THE COVID-19 ERA

The effect of the severe acute respiratory syndrome coronavirus 2 [(SARS-CoV-2), or COVID-19] pandemic and the relaxation of reimbursement and HIPAA regulations have led to the widespread utilization of telehealth in both rural and non-rural America. Before the pandemic, the health care system, overall, was experiencing relatively modest increases in telehealth from one year to the next. On March 6, 2020, Section 1135 waivers of the Social Security Act and the Coronavirus Preparedness and Response Supplemental Appropriations Act permitted Medicare to pay for telehealth visits from providers including doctors, nurse practitioners, psychologists, and social workers to include visits in a patient's place of residence (Centers for Medicare and Medicaid Services, 2020). The Centers for Medicare and Medicaid Services (CMS) encouraged the States' use of telehealth services across all of the populations served by Medicaid. States were encouraged to review services not traditionally offered via telehealth to identify methods by which those services could also be delivered via telehealth (Badaracco, n.d.).

These temporary measures issued by the Centers for Medicare and Medicaid Services (CMS) significantly expanded the list of covered telehealth services to also include:

- *Visits to Emergency Departments*
- *Virtual Home Health Care Visits*
- *Virtual Chiropractic Therapeutic Visits*
- *Virtual Physical Therapy, Occupational Therapy, Speech/Hearing Therapy*
- *Group Psychotherapy*
- *Eye Exams*
- *Virtual Autism Spectrum Disorder Therapy and Skills Training*
- *Physician's Weekly Radiation Treatment Management, and*
- *Acute Nursing Facility Care* (Centers for Medicare and Medicaid Services, n.d.) *CMS, 2020).*

As of February 2021, blanket waivers were still in place "through the end of the emergency declaration," with a retroactive effective date of March 1, 2020 (Centers for Medicare and Medicaid Services, 2020). Figure 3 displays the significant increase in telehealth visits from 2019 to 2020:

Figure 3. Increase in Claim Lines from 2019 to 2020

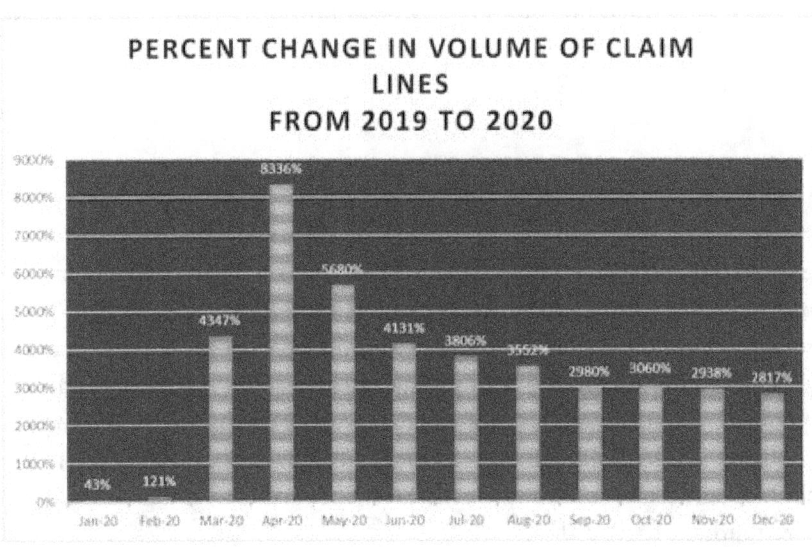

From December of 2019 to December of 2020, Telehealth claim line volume increased by 2,816.77 percent (A claim line is an individual service or procedure listed on an insurance claim). The frequency of the top five procedure codes by utilization increased in established patient office or other outpatient visits and psychotherapy and decreased in patient education and training and new patient visits. During the height of the pandemic transition to telehealth in April 2020, the increase in telehealth claim lines represented an increase of 8,335.51%. Since that time, telehealth visits have plateaued to an average of between six and 6.5% of total claim lines. It is noteworthy that telehealth diagnoses for mental health conditions increased more than forty-six percent and influenza and pneumonia, urinary tract infections, and eye infections dropped from the list of top five telehealth diagnoses from December 2019 to December 2020 (Fair Health, Inc., 2020). These trends are notable since they suggest a marked increase in COVID-19 related mental health needs and a reduction in non-emergent care. These changes are limited to telehealth visits only and do not, necessarily, reflect changes in claim lines for in-person visits which experienced a decline in overall visits of as much as 53.4% during March and April of 2020 with decreasing claim lines continuing through November of 2020, though to a lesser extent. The patterns of increased mental health claim lines and decreased medical claim lines continued throughout the study period. (FAIR Health, 2021).

Although telehealth was essential in mitigating distance and access challenges for all, the reliance on virtual connections during this incredible transition to telehealth, unintentionally served to increase health disparities for those without adequate access to the broadband required, including many in rural populations (Hirko, et al., 2020). However, with the increase in providers trained to use telehealth modalities and the increase in facilities building telehealth infrastructures, specialty services have become more accessible, creating long-term positive implications for those rural populations (Nagata, 2020).

QUALITY

Concern as to the quality of telemedicine compared with in-person visits spurred various research studies and encouraged the gathering, and assessment of, data to discern whether quality might suffer. In 2017, well before the COVID-19 pandemic, surveys and research suggested strong satisfaction responses, returns on investment of 10 percent or more, and an indication that patients planned to continue utilizing telehealth options. Virtually all surveys identified challenges with legal, regulatory, and reimbursement issues as limiting factors in the further development of telehealth (Foley & Lardner, LLP, 2017).

In 2019, AHRQ systematically reviewed 233 studies that each evaluated the effectiveness of telehealth consultations and found that telehealth either improved or produced equivalent clinical outcomes to in-person care (Totten, et al., 2019). An analysis of telemedicine in the orthopedic setting indicated high support by physicians for this method as a replacement for in-person visits and a belief that telemedicine was appropriate in 78.4% of the encounters. 92.9% of patients indicated they would use telemedicine again (Andrew M. Rizzi, 2020).

In a 2020 article on the efficacy of telemedicine during and after the COVID-19 pandemic, authors felt that the pandemic itself would provide a boost to telemedicine use in the immediate future, but that more robust long-term data on efficacy, safety, and health economics were necessary. They pointed out that the urological literature indicated a successful implementation in the management of prostate cancer (PCa), urinary incontinence (UI), Pelvic Organ Prolapse (POP), uncomplicated urinary stones, and uncomplicated urinary tract infections (UTIs) (Giacomo Novara, 2020).

In a study evaluating the use of telemedicine to screen Emergency Department (ED) patients, the efficiency between in-person screeners and telescreens was neither clinically relevant nor statistically significant once the telescreen methods became habitual. Further, the rate of patients who left without being seen (LWBS) decreased from 25.1% to 4.5% during certain hours when in-person screening was not traditionally available, and no difference in standards of care was noted (Nicholas James Rademacher, 2019).

LEGAL QUESTIONS

In the early 2000s when telehealth was primarily used to reach patients in rural areas, there was uncertainty related to legal questions it presented, such as those related to autonomy, confidentiality, licensure, and jurisdiction. It was thought that these unresolved legal issues would stunt telehealth's potential to increase access to care and would act as obstacles that had to be resolved before we would see the widespread adoption of telehealth throughout rural America and beyond. (Poe, 2000).

AUTONOMY

Autonomous decision-making, such as when a patient provides informed consent to medical treatment, requires that the provider explain risks, benefits, and reasonable alternatives that allow the patient to make an independent decision. With the increase in the use of telehealth, using varying modalities and technology, individual states revamped policies and regulations to ensure that patients were still making informed decisions. As of Fall 2020, 41 states and Washington, D.C. had telehealth consent requirements in either the Medicaid policy, law, or regulation (Center for Connected Health Policy, 2020). The Agency for Healthcare Research and Quality (AHRQ) offers resources that guide medical providers with respect to obtaining and documenting telehealth consent, including a consent form template for providers to use even when it is not required by the state (Agency for Healthcare Research and Quality, 2020).

CONFIDENTIALITY

The HIPAA Privacy Rule, first implemented in 1996, safeguards Protected Health Information (PHI), which includes all forms of "individually identifiable health information that relates to the past, present, or future physical or mental health or condition of an individual, the provision of health care to an individual, or the past, present, or future payment for the provision of health care to an individual" (Centers for Disease Control and Prevention, 2018). A subset of the Privacy Rule, The HIPAA Security Rule, applies to Electronic Protected Health Information (e-PHI), which includes all individually identifiable "health information a covered entity creates, receives, maintains, or transmits in electronic form (Centers for Disease Control and Prevention, 2018)."

In 2013, the Office for Civil Rights (OCR) in DHHS determined that although it might be unduly burdensome for some entities, to protect health information, patients had to be informed of potential risks associated with unencrypted email (Office for Civil Rights, Department of Health and Human Services p. 5634, 2013). Now, we commonly use technology that has the potential to make the risks even greater. For example, remote patient monitoring systems (RPM), that rely on the interaction of multiple devices and external entities, can expose health providers and patients to security and privacy risks at several different points in the process. (National Institute of Standards and Technology, 2020).

An RPM system collects biometric data from the patient at a remote location, such as the home, and sends the data back to the clinical team, often using a third-party vendor as the telehealth platform provider. To enable organizations to identify areas where processes can be strengthened to improve privacy The National Institute of Standards and Technology of the U.S. Department of Commerce (NIST) released the NIST Privacy Framework tool through enterprise risk management. (National Institute of Standards and Technology, 2020). From its release in January 2020 to January 2021 the NIST framework was downloaded 31,000 times and in more than 10 countries (Lefkovitz, 2021).

The Health Information Technology for Economic and Clinical Health Act (HITECH Act) was created, as part of the American Recovery and Investment Act by President Obama, in 2009 to encourage wider adoption of electronic health records (EHRs). Rural areas lagged in the adoption, in part due to problems related to insufficient broadband and internet access. Additionally, disparities in the use of the internet may have contributed to the slow adoption (National Rural Health Association, 2017).

In 2013, the requirements of HITECH were incorporated into HIPAA when the Department of Health and Human Services modified HIPAA enforcement rules (Office for Civil Rights, Department of Health and Human Services, 2013). The revisions to the enforcement rules also served to increase flexibility and reduce burden, but to ensure informed consent. For example, providers could send patients unencrypted emails "if [the providers] advised the individual of the risk, and the individual still [preferred] the unencrypted email" (Office for Civil Rights, Department of Health and Human Services p. 5634, 2013).

PHYSICIAN LICENSING AND OUT-OF-STATE PRACTICE

Although physicians licensing is granted by a particular state, there are scenarios where treatment by out-of-state physicians occurs regularly. This may arise via consultation with an existing patient who travels out of the state, where a physician consults with an out-of-state specialist or other medical providers (HealthIT.gov, 2019), as well as via interstate licensing compacts (Interstate Medical Licensure Compact, 2020). During the COVID-19 Public Health Emergency, several U.S. States and Territories modified requirements to allow licensure waivers. As of November 20, 2020, 40 U.S. States, along with Guam, The Commonwealth of the Northern Mariana Islands, and Puerto Rico recognized some type of waiver. Washington, D.C., and 36 States expedited licensure for inactive and retired licensees (Federation of State Medical Boards, 2018).

JURISDICTION

Where can a telemedicine medical malpractice case be filed if the medical provider lives in a different state than the patient? Telemedicine often crosses state lines, so deciphering jurisdictional issues is vital. Most states allow the patient to file the case in the state where the patient lives or where the doctor's office is located but some states, such as North Carolina, demand that telemedicine medical malpractice cases filed by a resident must be brought within that state (Medical Justice, 2016).

There could still be Choice of Law issues, however, if it is unclear as to whether the law from the patient's state or the provider's state governs the action (The National Law Review, 2019).

Any unresolved jurisdictional questions will make it difficult for insurance carriers to assess potential risks (The National Law Review, 2019). Malpractice policies vary and can differ by area of specialty. Physicians cannot assume that medical treatments performed in person will automatically be covered by a medical malpractice insurance policy. Depending on the policy, however, telemedicine malpractice may be covered. Providers may also consider securing cyber liability insurance to cover certain incidents such as data breaches.

GLOBAL TELEHEALTH IN THE COVID-19 ERA

During the onset of the COVID-19 pandemic, the World Health Organization in coordination with national health organizations recognized the value of telemedicine and telehealth to reduce the risk of transmission, especially in the United Kingdom, the United States, China, and Australia, and a framework of telemedicine was developed to utilize telemedicine when addressing the needs of both asymptomatic and symptomatic patients. Under the framework, patients would receive care according to the severity of the symptoms using remote monitoring if symptoms were not severe; teleconsultation for patients with mild symptoms, and emergency medical care for severe symptoms. The post-release follow-up would include telespecialist interaction for mild cases; teleradiology for hospitalized and ICU patients and tele-ICU care when required (Ohannessian, Duong, & Odone, 2020).

Most countries did not have the regulatory framework at the onset of the pandemic and had to create emergency authorizations to permit and reimburse the delivery of care to patients. Relaxation of privacy protections also presented a challenge to permit the utilization of mostly free video chat programs in violation of most data security protocols to be used to decrease the risk of disease transmission. Countries like Italy, with one of the highest incidences of COVID-19, did not have a mechanism for telemedicine in its National Health Service. During the pandemic, the Ministry of Health allowed reimbursement of teleconsultations and teleexpertise under the National Health Insurance for COVID-19 symptomatic patients without a previously established relationship with the provider (including physicians, nurses, midwives, and speech therapists (Ohannessian, et al., 2020).

In April of 2020, Ethiopia achieved a Google search popularity score of 100 (out of 100) followed by the United States at 59 for the same month during a month that experienced a telemedicine search query jump of 525% (The Evolving Enterprise, 2020). This statistic speaks favorably for a country where 85% of its population lives in remote locations and would benefit from the implementation of telehealth initiatives. Between 2004 and 2006 a pilot project involving 20 physicians tested a telemedicine system with some level of success. They utilized teledermatology, teleradiology, and telepathology and concluded a demonstrated practical applicability despite its premature phase of development (Shiferaw & Zolfo, 2012).

THE FUTURE OF TELEHEALTH

The Health Resources and Services Administration (HRSA) is the agency of the U.S. Department of Health and Human Services dedicated to improving health outcomes of, and addressing health disparities related to, those in remote areas as well as those who are economically or medically vulnerable, uninsured, or enrolled in Medicare (Health Resources & Services Administration, 2021). The HRSA works to increase and improve the use of telehealth to meet the needs of these underserved populations (Dinesen, 2016).

The Federal Office of Rural Health Policy (FORHP), under the HRSA umbrella, supports rural health programs, including veterans' rural health access programs and rural health networks (Federal Office of Rural Health Policy, 2017). Through the Office for the Advancement of Telehealth (OAT), the FORHP funds programs, provides resources, and promotes the use of telehealth technologies for healthcare delivery and education (Health Resources & Services Administration, 2021).

Whether the utilization of telehealth and telemedicine will return to the pre-COVID-19 levels or maintain its current level is unknown. Fair Health noted a reduction in telehealth visits following a peak in April 2020. Certainly, new, unanticipated avenues for virtual treatment, communication, and health administration will have been identified and used if legislative authorization for reimbursement continues.

Incentives to invest in telehealth should improve as reimbursement moves to a value-based pay model (Dinesen, 2016). Most outpatient visits can be triaged to telemedicine without compromising health or quality; The infrastructure already existed and was enhanced by the move to electronic health records; logistics, including training and staffing, can be put in place fairly easily; and, this can all be accomplished with minimal disruption and resistance (Bashshur, 2020).

Health systems have developed bots that connect higher-risk patients to nurse triage and may direct lower-risk patients to make an appointment for a future visit and use built-in automated screening algorithms for the intake process (Hollander & Carr, 2020). Some health systems use electronic intensive care unit (e-ICU) monitoring programs that are ideal for monitoring sicker patients and allow clinicians to monitor as many as 100 patients remotely (Hollander & Carr, 2020).

One of the trends worth noting is the elimination of the no-cost sharing benefit that was extended by both Anthem and UnitedHealthcare insurers during the COVID-19 pandemic. In October of 2020, several of them announced plans to reimplement copays, coinsurance, and deductible charges for virtual visits which are not related to COVID-19 (Healthcare Financial Management Association, 2020). Following this announcement, Aetna will end its $0 copay for specialist telehealth and mental health counseling visits on January 31, 2020 (Aetna, 2021). Medicare has treated telehealth services in the same manner as in-person visits with patient responsibility at 20% of the Medicare-approved amount for doctor and other health care provider services and the Part B deductible applies (Agency for Healthcare Research and Quality, 2020). In 2020, Medicare expanded services to include renal dialysis facilities and at home, emergency department visits at home, in-home physical and occupational therapy, visits delivered by audio-only devices, and virtual check-ins and E-visits (Medicare.gov, 2021). However, in March of 2020, the Department of Health and Human Services Office of the Inspector General issued a policy that permits physicians or other practitioners to reduce or waive coinsurance and deductibles without the potential to implicate the Federal anti-kickback statute as long as the telehealth services are furnished during the Covid-19 Public Health Emergency Declaration (DHHS Office of Inspector General, 2020).

In early December of 2020, the 2021 Medicare Physician Fee Schedule (MPFS) was released by CMS which includes new telehealth services that can be reimbursed under Category 1, making coverage permanent beyond the conclusion of the Public Health Emergency (PHE). These additions include:

- Group Psychotherapy (CPT code 90853);
- Psychological and Neuropsychological Testing (CPT code 96121);
- Domiciliary, Rest Home, or Custodial Care services;
- Established patients (CPT codes 99334-99335);
- Home Visits, Established Patient (CPT codes 99347-99348);
- Cognitive Assessment and Care Planning Services (CPT code 99483);
- Visit Complexity Inherent to Certain Office/Outpatient Evaluation and Management (E/M) (HCPCS code G2211); and,Prolonged Services (HCPCS code G2212).

CMS expanded the list of care providers using telehealth to include clinical social workers, clinical psychologists, physical and occupational therapists, and speech-language pathologists. Additionally, CMS will cover one nursing facility telehealth visit every 14, instead of the previous 30 days. Other Category 3 services have been included in the PFE which will be reimbursed until the end of the year in which the public health emergency concludes (Wicklund, 2020).

In a press release accompanying the Physician Fee Schedule, CMS noted that only 15,000 fee-for-service beneficiaries per week had received a Medicare telemedicine service before the Public Health Emergency. That number increased to show that 24.5 million out of 63 million received a telemedicine service from mid-March until mid-October. They also announced the commission of a study of new opportunities for telehealth and virtual care supervision, and remote monitoring can be used (CMS.gov, 2020).

The Covid-19 public health emergency has resulted in devastating losses in life and significant challenges to the entire global healthcare systems. In the United States, the adoption of 1135 waivers have permitted the expansion of telehealth to serve patients throughout the country. Congress and state governments are under pressure to examine the emergency measures, to expand upon the telehealth options, and to make them permanent. It is clear that telehealth has been very effective during the Public Health Emergency of the COVID-19 pandemic and both providers and patients would like to see its continuation.

Figure 4. Test Your Knowledge

Test Your Knowledge of Telehealth Terminology		
Asynchronous	Medicare	Store and Forward
Claim Line	Physician Fee Schedule	Synchronous
Electronic Health Records	Protected Health Information	Telehealth
Eligible Originating Sites	Remote Patient Monitoring	Telehealth Consent Forms
Health Disparities	Rural Health	Telemedicine
Medicaid	Section 1135 Waivers	

REFERENCES

Ackerman, B. G. (2019, April 17). Is the Doctor In? Medical Malpractice Issues in the Age of Telemedicine. *The National Law Review*. https://www.natlawreview.com/article/doctor-medical-malpractice-issues-age-telemedicine

Aetna. (2021). *Get started with telemedicine*. Aetna. https://www.aetna.com/individuals-families/member-rights-resources/covid19/telemedicine.html

Agency for Healthcare Research and Quality. (2020, October). *CAHPS Health Plan Survey*. AHRQ. https://www.ahrq.gov/cahps/surveys-guidance/hp/index.html

Agency for Healthcare Research and Quality. (2020, September). *How to Obtain Consent for Telehealth*. AHRQ. https://www.ahrq.gov/health-literacy/improve/informed-consent/obtain.html

Andriola, M. (2019). Telemedicine and Legal Disruption. *Health Law & Policy Brief, 13*(2), [iii]-30. https://heinonline.org/HOL/P?h=hein.journals/heallaw13&i=73

Aronson, S. H. (1977). The Lancet on the Telephone 1876-1975. *Medical History, 21*(1), 69–87. doi:10.1017/S0025727300037182 PMID:320411

Badaracco, A. (n.d.). *Medicaid State Plan Fee-for-Service Payments for Services Delivered Via Telehealth*. Medicaid. https://www.medicaid.gov/medicaid/benefits/downloads/medicaid-telehealth-services.pdf

Bashshur, R. e., Doarn, C. R., Frenk, J. M., Kvedar, J. C., & Woolliscroft, J. O. (2020). Telemedicine and the COVID-19 Pandemic, Lessons for the Future. *Telemedicine Journal and e-Health, 26*(5), 571–573. doi:10.1089/tmj.2020.29040.rb PMID:32275485

Baumann, P. K., & Scales, T. (2016). *History of Information Communication Technology and Telehealth*. Winston-Salem State University. https://search-proquest-com.courseinfo.wssu.edu/docview/1863562170?pq-origsite=summon

Berg, J. (2014). The E-Health Revolution and the Necessary Evolution of Informed Consent. *Indiana Health Law Review*. https://heinonline.org/HOL/P?h=hein.journals/inhealr11&i=597

Board on Health Care Services. (2012, November 20). *The Role of Telehealth in an Evolving Health Care Environment: Workshop Summary*. Institute of Medicine. https://www.ncbi.nlm.nih.gov/books/NBK207141/#_NBK207141_pubdet_

Bortniker, F., & Warren, A. (2020, April 15). *COVID-19: Resources for Oncology Providers (Telehealth, Clinical Trials, Reporting Deadlines)*. Winston-Salem State University. https://search-proquest-com.courseinfo.wssu.edu/docview/2389842056/126488F7309143FEPQ/3?accountid=15070

Center for Connected Health Policy. (2020). *State Telehealth Laws & Reimbursement Policies*. CCHPCA. https://www.cchpca.org/sites/default/files/2020-10/CCHP%2050%20STATE%20REPORT%20FALL%202020%20FINAL.pdf

Centers for Disease Control and Prevention. (2018, September 14). *Health Insurance Portability and Accountability Act of 1996 (HIPAA)*. CDC. https://www.cdc.gov/phlp/publications/topic/hipaa.html

Centers for Disease Control and Prevention. (2019). *Health Insurance Portability and Accountability Act of 1996 (HIPAA)*. CDC. https://www.cdc.gov/phlp/publications/topic/hipaa.html

Centers for Medicare and Medicaid Services. (2020, February 19). *COVID-19 Emergency Declaration Blanket Waivers for Health Care Providers.* CMS. https://www.cms.gov/files/document/covid-19-emergency-declaration-waivers.pdf

Centers for Medicare and Medicaid Services. (2020, March 17). *Medicare Telemedicine Health Care Provider Fact Sheet.* CMS. https://www.cms.gov/newsroom/fact-sheets/medicare-telemedicine-health-care-provider-fact-sheet

Centers for Medicare and Medicaid Services. (2020). *Rural Health Council.* CMS. https://www.cms.gov/About-CMS/Agency-Information/OMH/equity-initiatives/rural-health/rural-health-council

Centers for Medicare and Medicaid Services. (n.d.). *List of Telehealth Services.* CMS. https://www.cms.gov/Medicare/Medicare-General-Information/Telehealth/Telehealth-Codes

Christensen, C. (2012). *Disruptive Innovation.* Clayton Christensen. https://claytonchristensen.com/key-concepts/

Christensen, C. M. (2011). *Disrupting College.* Center for American Progress: https://www.americanprogress.org/issues/economy/reports/2011/02/08/9034/disrupting-college/

Christensen, C. M. (2015, December 1). What Is Disruptive Innovation? *Harvard Business Review.* https://hbr.org/2015/12/what-is-disruptive-innovation

CMS.gov. (2020, October 28). *Rural Health Council.* CMS. https://www.cms.gov/About-CMS/Agency-Information/OMH/equity-initiatives/rural-health/rural-health-council

CMS.gov. (2020, December 1). *Trump Administration Finalizes Permanent Expansion of Medicare Telehealth Services and Improved Payment for Time Doctors Spend with Patients.* CMS. https://www.cms.gov/newsroom/press-releases/trump-administration-finalizes-permanent-expansion-medicare-telehealth-services-and-improved-payment

Department of Health and Human Services Office of Inspector General. (2018, April). *CMS Paid Practitioners for Telehealth Services That Did Not Meet Medicare Requirements.* Garner Health News. http://garnerhealth.com/wp-content/uploads/2014/02/51600058.pdf

DHHS Office of Inspector General. (2020, March 17). *OIG Policy Statement Regarding Physicians and Other Practitioners That Reduce or Waive Amounts Owed by Federal Health Care Program Beneficiaries for Telehealth Services During the 2019 Novel Coronavirus (COVID-19) Outbreak.* OIG. https://oig.hhs.gov/fraud/docs/alertsandbulletins/2020/policy-telehealth-2020.pdf

Dinesen, B. e., Nonnecke, B., Lindeman, D., Toft, E., Kidholm, K., Jethwani, K., Young, H. M., Spindler, H., Oestergaard, C. U., Southard, J. A., Gutierrez, M., Anderson, N., Albert, N. M., Han, J. J., & Nesbitt, T. (2016). Personalized Telehealth in the Future: A Global Research Agenda. *Journal of Medical Internet Research, 18*(3), e53. doi:10.2196/jmir.5257 PMID:26932229

eVisit. (2021). *History of Telemedicine*. eVisit. https://evisit.com/resources/history-of-telemedicine/

Fair Health, Inc. (2020). *States by the Numbers*. Fair Health. https://www.fairhealth.org/states-by-the-numbers/telehealth

Federal Office of Rural Health Policy. (2017). *Official web site of the U.S. Health Resources & Services Administration*. Health Resources and Services Administration. https://www.hrsa.gov/rural-health/index.html

Federation of State Medical Boards. (2018). *Covid-19*. FSMB. https://www.fsmb.org/advocacy/covid-19/

Fisher, M. (2020, March 19). *Covid-19's Impact on Telehealth & HIPAA Regulations.* Winston-Salem State University. https://search-proquest-com.courseinfo.wssu.edu/docview/2379060880?pq-origsite=summon

Foley & Lardner. LLP. (2017). *2017 Telemedicine and Digital Health Survey.* Foley. https://www.foley.com/en/files/uploads/2017-Telemedicine-Survey-Report-11-8-17.pdf

Foley & Lardner. LLP. (2021). *Telehealth21 Summit Virtual Conference.* Foley. https://www.foley.com/en/insights/events/2021/03/telehealth21-summit-virtual-conference

Health, F. A. I. R. (2021, March 2). The Impact of COVID-19 on Pediatric Mental Health. *Fair Health.* https://s3.amazonaws.com/media2.fairhealth.org/whitepaper/asset/The%20Impact%20of%20COVID-19%20on%20Pediatric%20Mental%20Health%20-%20A%20Study%20of%20Private%20Healthcare%20Claims%20-%20A%20FAIR%20Health%20White%20Paper.pdf

Health IT gov. (2019, April 15). *Are there state licensing issues related to telehealth?* The Office of the National Coordinator for Health Information Teaching. https://www.healthit.gov/faq/are-there-state-licensing-issues-related-telehealth

Health Resources & Services Administration. (2021, January). *Telehealth Programs.* HRSA. https://www.hrsa.gov/rural-health/telehealth

Healthcare Financial Management Association. (2020, October 7). *Major insurers roll back no-cost sharing telehealth services.* HFMA. https://www.hfma.org/topics/technology/article/-major-insurers-roll-back-no-cost-sharing-telehealth-services.html

Hirko, K. A., Kerver, J. M., Ford, S., Szafranski, C., Beckett, J., Kitchen, C., & Wendling, A. L. (2020). Telehealth in response to the COVID-19 pandemic: Implications for rural health disparities. [Retrieved from https://doi.org/10.1093/jamia/ocaa156]. *Journal of the American Medical Informatics Association, 27*(11), 1816–1818.

Hollander, J., & Carr, B. (2020). Virtually Perfect?? Telemedicine for COVID-19. *New England Journal of Medicine, 382*https://doi.org/10.1056/NEJMp2003539 doi:.

Hwang, C. J., & Lappan, C. M. (2014). Utilization of Telemedicine in the U.S. Military in a Deployed Setting. *Military Medicine*, *179*, 1347–1353.

Interstate Medical Licensure Compact. (2020). *A Faster Pathway to Physician Licensure.* IMLCC. https://www.imlcc.org/

Journal, H. I. P. A. A. (2018). *What is the HITECH Act?* Retrieved November 29, 2020, from https://www.hipaajournal.com/what-is-the-hitech-act/

Journal, H. I. P. A. A. (2014-2020). *What is the HITECH Act.* Retrieved November 29, 2020, from https://www.hipaajournal.com/what-is-the-hitech-act/

Lefkovitz, N. (2021, January 14). *Happy First Birthday, NIST Privacy Framework!* NIST. https://www.nist.gov/blogs/cybersecurity-insights/happy-first-birthday-nist-privacy-framework

Maheu, M., & Whitten, P. Allen, & Ace. (2002). E-Health, Telehealth, and Telemedicine: A Guide to Startup and Success. John Wiley & Sons.

Mathematica. (2020, November 23). *Maintaining Flexible Telehealth Policies After COVID-19.* Retrieved November 25, 2020, from https://www.mathematica.org/our-publications-and-findings/publications/maintaining-flexible-telehealth-policies-after-covid-19

Mayo Clinic. (2020). *Managing your health in the age of Wi-Fi.* Retrieved November 29, 2020, from https://www.mayoclinic.org/healthy-lifestyle/consumer-health/in-depth/telehealth/art-20044878

Mayo Clinic. (2020, May 15). *Telehealth: Technology meets health care.* Retrieved November 28, 2020, from https://www.mayoclinic.org/healthy-lifestyle/consumer-health/in-depth/telehealth/art-20044878

Medical Justice. (2016, August 12). *Liability in Telemedicine: "Can you sue me now?".* Retrieved March 15, 2021, from https://medicaljustice.com/liability-telemedicine-can-sue-now/

Medicare.gov. (2021). *Telehealth.* Medicare. https://www.medicare.gov/coverage/telehealth

Nagata, J. M. (2020). Rapid Scale-Up of Telehealth During the COVID-19 Pandemicand Implications for Subspecialty Care in Rural Areas. *The Journal of Rural Health.* doi:10.1111/jrh.12433

National Institute of Standards and Technology. (2020, January 16). *NIST Privacy Framework: A Tool for Improving Privacy Through Enterprise Risk Management, Version 1.0.* NIST. https://nvlpubs.nist.gov/nistpubs/CSWP/NIST.CSWP.01162020.pdf

National Rural Health Association. (2017, February). A Rural-Urban Comparison of Hospitals Participating in the Medicare Electronic Health Record Incentive Program. *Rural Health.* https://www.ruralhealthweb.org/NRHA/media/Emerge_NRHA/Advocacy/Policy%20documents/Medicare-Electronic-Health_Feb-2017_NRHA-Policy-Paper.pdf

NEJM Catalyst. (2018, February 1). Innovations in Care Delivery. *New England Journal of Medicine.* https://catalyst.nejm.org/doi/full/10.1056/CAT.18.0268

New York State Department of Health. (2021). *Foreign Countries with Universal Health Care.* NYSDH. https://www.health.ny.gov/regulations/hcra/univ_hlth_care.htm

Nguyen, C. M. (2020). Reduction in Medical Evacuations from Iraq and Syria Following Introduction of an Asynchronous Telehealth System. *Military Medicine, 185*(9-10), 1693–1699.

Nicholas James Rademacher, M. G. (2019). Use of Telemedicine to Screen Patients in the Emergency Department: Matched Cohort Study Evaluating Efficiency and Patient Safety of Telemedicine. *JMIR Medical Informatics, 7*(2).

Novak, M. (2012, March 14). Telemedicine Predicted in 1925. *Smithsonian Magazine.* https://www.smithsonianmag.com/history/telemedicine-predicted-in-1925-124140942/

Novara, G. C. (2020). Telehealth in Urology: A systematic review of the literature. How much can telemedicine be useful during and after the Covid-19 Pandemic? *European Urology.*

Office for Civil Rights. (2013, January 25). Modifications to the HIPAA Privacy, Security, Enforcement, and Breach Notification Rules Under the Health Information Technology for Economic and Clinical Health Act and the Genetic Information Nondiscrimination Act; Other Modifications to the HIPAA Rules. *Department of Health and Human Services,* p. 5634. https://www.federalregister.gov/documents/2013/01/25/2013-01073/modifications-to-the-hipaa-privacy-security-enforcement-and-breach-notification-rules-under-the

Office of the National Coordinator for Health Information Technology. (2016, November). *Federal Telehealth Compendium.* Federal Office of Rural Health Policy. https://mtelehealth.com/wp-content/uploads/2019/10/Federal-Telehealth-Compendium.pdf

Ohannessian, R., Duong, T., & Odone, A. (2020). Global Telemedicine Implementation and Integration Within Health Systems to Fight the COVID-19 Pandemic: A Call to Action. *JMIR Public Health and Surveillannce, 6*(2).

Poe, K. (2000). Telemedicine Liability: Texas and Other States Delve into the Uncertainties of Health Care Delivery via Advanced Communications Technology. *Review of Litigation, 20*(3), 681–708. https://heinonline.org/HOL/P?h=hein.journals/rol20&i=699

Rizzi, A. M. (2020, September 16). The new ‘normal’: Rapid adoption of telemedicine in orthopaedics during the COVID-19 pandemic. *Injury.*

Shiferaw, F., & Zolfo, M. (2012, April 2). The role of information communication technology (ICT) towards universal health coverage: the first steps of a telemedicine project in Ethiopia. *Global Health Action, 5.* https://www.ncbi.nlm.nih.gov/pmc/articles/PMC3318899/

Simpson, A. T., Doarn, C. R., & Garber, S. J. (2020). Interagency Cooperation in the Twilight of the Great Society: Telemedicine, NASA, and the Papago Nation. *Journal of Policy History, 32*(1), 25–51. doi:10.1017/S0898030619000265

Stein, M. M. (2020, 03 11). *Coronavirus Funding Package Waives Medicare Telehealth Restrictions.* Winston-Salem State University. https://search-proquest-com.courseinfo.wssu.edu/docview/2375735192?pq-origsite=summon

TeleHealth Access for Seniors. (n.d.). *TeleHealth Access*. TeleHealth Access for Seniors. https://www.telehealthforseniors.org/

The Evolving Enterprise. (2020, April 24). *Telemedicine search queries jump by 525%, Ethiopia ranks highest.* The Evolving Enterprise. https://www.theee.ai/2020/04/24/2038-telemedicine-search-queries-jump-by-525-ethiopia-ranks-highest/

The Office of the National Coordinator for Health Information Technology (ONC). (2019, October 17). *What is telehealth? How is telehealth different from telemedicine?* HRSA. https://www.healthit.gov/faq/what-telehealth-how-telehealth-different-telemedicine

Totten, A., Hansen, R., Wagner, J., Stillman, L., Ivlev, I., Davis-O'Reilly, C., & McDonagh, M. (2019). Telehealth for Acute and Chronic Care Consultations. *Europe PMC.* https://europepmc.org/article/NBK/nbk547239

UNC School of Medicine. (2020, January 2). *The Ultimate Telemedicine: UNC Expert Helps Treat Astronaut's Blood Clot During NASA Mission.* Retrieved November 29, 2020, from https://news.unchealthcare.org/2020/01/telemedicine-astronauts-blood-clot-nasa/

U.S. Department of Health and Human Services. (2020, May 07). *HIPAA flexibility during DOVID-19.* HHS. https://www.hhs.gov/coronavirus/telehealth/index.html

U.S. Department of Veterans Affairs. (2020). *Office of Rural Health*. DVA. https://www.ruralhealth.va.gov/aboutus/programs.asp

U.S. Health Resources & Services Administration. (2017). *About HRSA*. HRSA. https://www.hrsa.gov/about/index.htm

U.S. Health Resources & Services Administration. (2017). *Federal Office of Rural Health Policy*. HRSA. https://www.hrsa.gov/rural-health/index.html

U.S. Health Resources & Services Administration. (2017). *Telehealth Programs*. HRSA. https://www.hrsa.gov/rural-health/telehealth

Wallut, L., Peyron, C., Hervieu-Bègue, M., Osseby, G.-V., Giroud, M., Legris, N., ... Lejeune, C. (2020, April). Efficiency of telemedicine for acute stroke: A cost-effectiveness analysis from a French pilot study. *International Journal of Technology Assessment in Health Care, 36*(2), 126–132.

Wicklund, E. (2020, December 2). CMS Finalizes Telehealth, RPM Coverage in 2021 Physician Fee Schedule. *mHealth Intelligence.* https://mhealthintelligence.com/news/cms-finalizes-telehealth-rpm-coverage-in-2021-physician-fee-schedule

Wicklund, E. (2020, January 2). NASA Uses Telehealth to Answer a Space Station Medical Emergency. *mHealth Intelligence.* https://mhealthintelligence.com/news/nasa-uses-telehealth-to-answer-a-space-station-medical-emergency

Wicklund, E. (2021, March 29). New Bills Target Telehealth Coverage for Substance Abuse, Mental Health Services. *mHealth Intelligence.* https://mhealthintelligence.com/news/new-bills-target-telehealth-coverage-for-substance-abuse-mental-health-services

Wong, M. Y., Gunasekeran, D. V., Nusinovici, S., Sabanayagam, C., Yeo, K. K., Cheng, C.-Y., & Tham, Y.-C. (2021). Telehealth Demand Trends During the COVID-19 Pandemic in the Top 50 Most Affected Countries: Infodemiological Evaluation. *JMIR Public Health and Surveillance*, *7*(2).

World Health Organization. (2016). *Telehealth: Analysis of third global survey on eHeallth based on the reported data by countries, 2016.* WHO. https://www.who.int/gho/goe/telehealth/en/

APPENDIX: ADDITIONAL STUDENT RESOURCES/LINKS

1. Telehealth Consent Form:
   a. Internet Citation: AHRQ's Easy-to-Understand Telehealth Consent Form. Content last reviewed September 2020. Agency for Healthcare Research and Quality, Rockville, MD. https://www.ahrq.gov/health-literacy/improve/informed-consent/index.html
2. CAHPS Quality Survey Tools:
   a. Internet Citation: Principles Underlying CAHPS Surveys. Content last reviewed January 2020. Agency for Healthcare Research and Quality, Rockville, MD. https://www.ahrq.gov/cahps/about-cahps/principles/index.html
3. Non-profit Telehealth Access for Seniors and Low-income communities
   a. Provide resources, including devices, instruction, tech support. https://www.telehealthforseniors.org/
4. The Center for Connected Health Policy – The National Telehealth Policy Resource Center
   a. Includes current state laws and policies; legislation tracking; and telehealth resources https://www.cchpca.org/
5. The National Consortium of Telehealth Resource Centers
   a. The National Consortium of Telehealth Resource Centers (NCTRC) is a collaborative of 12 regional and 2 national Telehealth Resource Centers (TRCs), committed to implementing telehealth programs for rural and underserved communities https://telehealthresourcecenter.org/

Chapter 7
The Shortage of Healthcare Workers in the United States:
A Call to Action

Jill JoAnn Harp
https://orcid.org/0000-0003-0845-0682
Winston-Salem State University, USA

ABSTRACT

This chapter discusses the current state of healthcare workers in the United States and strategies that show promise in mitigating shortages. Although some strategies involve leveraging technology, it is more important to provide students with an adequate science, technology, engineering, and mathematics (STEM) education prior to entering college. This would allow them to excel in the college level science classes needed to become doctors, nurses, mental healthcare professionals, physician assistants, etc., concomitant with mitigating the high attrition observed in these courses. In addition, diversity and inclusion efforts along with the invaluable role of historically black colleges and universities (HBCUs) will also be discussed.

INTRODUCTION

The strength of a nation's healthcare system is heavily dependent on having an adequate number of qualified individuals who receive a science education that prepares them for college-level math, biology, and chemistry. With math being a strong indicator of success in the latter two disciplines (Bryk & Triesman, 2010). Together, these courses serve as prerequisites for those entering allied health and science, technology, engineering, and math (STEM) programs. Globally our nation

DOI: 10.4018/978-1-6684-4060-5.ch007

ranks 22nd in math and 16th in science and although our healthcare workforce needs increase, the number of qualified students from K-12 through postsecondary school to fill this void, drastically decreases. Notably, our nation is in dire need of developing a more diverse workforce, especially as demographics change (Vespa & Armstrong, 2020). It is projected that 2030 will mark a transformation due to (1) growth in the US population to 350 million people, (2) increase in the Hispanic, African American, Biracial, and Asian populations and (3) net international migration of Asian populations. Without diversifying and growing our healthcare workforce, our nation's ability to address deleterious diseases and disorders while eliminating health disparities, continues to be in jeopardy. In addition, individuals over 65 are projected to grow to 21% of the population in 2030 and equal the number of youths under eighteen. Due to this increase, employment in healthcare occupations is projected to grow to 3.3 million by decade's end, much faster than the average for all occupations. Also, a substantial percentage of healthcare workers will need training to address geriatric needs. Lastly, the graying of America is co-occurring with mass retirements of Baby Boomers; as such, the healthcare profession may suffer immensely because the intellectual capital associated with the profession will leave with retirees. Hence, strategies to transfer best practices to the next generation of diverse, adequately prepared, culturally competent healthcare professionals are critical for optimal patient care.

This article discusses the current state of healthcare workers in the United States and strategies that show promise in mitigating shortages. Diversity and Inclusion efforts along with the invaluable role of HBCUs will also be discussed.

NUMBER OF HEALTHCARE PROFESSIONALS NEEDED

Physicians/Surgeons Shortage:

It is predicted by Kirch and Petelle (2017) that by 2030 there will be a shortage of approximately 121,000 physicians; this represents a national deficit of 139,160 physician jobs in the US (Kirch and Petelle, 2017). It is worth mentioning however, that this shortage is geographical (Zhang et al., 2020). Hence, the western US region is forecasted to have a physician shortage ratio (69 job shortage per 100,000 people), while the Northeast region will have a surplus (50 job excess per 100,000 people). The desire to provide optimal care is important to doctors. Due to the current shortage along with COVID-19 hospitalizations, several are at the brink of exhaustion (Reith, 2018; Nguyen, 2021). This leads to premature retirements or physicians opting to work less than full-time.

Nurses, Nurse Practitioners, and Physician Assistants Shortages

By 2030, there will be a national deficit of 918,232 registered nurses in the US (Juraschek et al., 2017; Alexander et al., 2021) and enrollment in nursing school programs is not keeping pace with the projected demand for nurses. Coupled with the limited slots available and the continued shortage of nursing school faculty available to teach in these programs led to the denial of 80,407 qualified applicants. As with other healthcare workers, nurses are nearing retirement (Mossberg, 2018) and retention becomes problematic when some face burnout due to understaffing (Castro et al., 2017). Burnout is known to cause subsequent reduced patient care (Reith, 2018).

Fortunately, there will be no shortage of nurse practitioners' (NP) in any state. However, unlike physicians and Physician Assistants (PAs), in many states, NPs are limited through scope of practice (SOP) regulations that impose restrictions on their ability to provide patient care. These regulations dictate the type and level of care they are allowed to provide by the state in which they are practicing. These were implemented to ensure quality of NP-delivered care due to differences in physician and NP training. However, recent research found no differences in quality of NP-delivered care across states regardless of SOP restrictions (Kurtzman et al., 2017; Kandrack et al., 2019).

For PAs, employment is projected to grow approximately 31% to 2029, much faster than the average for all occupations. Although there will be a shortage of PAs in the US, it is currently unknown which geographic areas will suffer the most and the extent of the shortage.

Mental Healthcare Worker Shortage

COVID-19 continues to take its toll on mental healthcare professionals (Kuriakose, 2020). Beginning in mid-March of 2020, those who were already suffering from mental disorders experienced increased stress and depression due to the increasing number of deaths in the US. In addition, mass unemployment cause individuals to be more stressed due to financial uncertainty and decrease in wages. The aforementioned, compounded with conflicting and oftentimes sobering media coverage, added to the stress individuals were experiencing (Holman et al., 2020). Hence, the COVID-19 outbreak placed more pressure on an already understaffed system. Indeed, frontline healthcare workers were also in increased need of mental health services. This is partly due to emotionally and physically caring for large numbers of infected individuals, shortage of Personal Protective Equipment (PPE), anxiety about getting infected and in turn, infecting loved ones, witnessing coworkers' infection, and sometimes death from the coronavirus (Ayanian, 2020).

MITIGATING THE SHORTAGE

Enabling Technologies

Telehealth (non-clinical), telemedicine (clinical), and telephonic visits have increased since March 2020 due to the desire to slow the spread of the coronavirus and to alleviate an already burdened healthcare system. Video visits have proven to be extremely valuable for non-urgent patient care. COVID-19 helped to normalize this practice and with the ability to transfer remote monitoring patient data, healthcare providers can give quality care without risking the spread of the coronavirus (Mann et al., 2020). Because of its lower cost and time effectiveness, the expanded use of telehealth is not likely to reverse to the pre-COVID era. This is especially advantageous for those in rural areas. In addition, the Center for Medicare and Medicaid Services (CMS) allows for full reimbursement for mental telehealth visits (Kichloo, 2020). Nonetheless, this is a temporary decision and may be reversed as the COVID-19 crisis abates (Lepkowsky, 2020).

Physicians/Surgeons

To offset physician shortages, steps can be taken to ensure they get the support needed and in turn, care for their patients with minimal to no burnout (Yates, 2020). Burnout must be addressed because it is connected to the likelihood of a physician making a major medical error when providing care and can also be associated with the quality of care received by the patient. Hence, supporting physicians' need for mental healthcare without attaching stigma and/or the threat of losing their license is ideal, receiving holistic appreciation from leadership, ensuring an infrastructure that minimizes administrative burden and allows for a healthy work-life balance, along with promoting efficient teams would allow for a more manageable profession (Thomas et al., 2018).

Nurses, Nurse Practitioners, and Physician Assistants

COVID-19 has increased awareness immensely regarding the need to address the shortage of nurses. On the federal level, The Department of Labor released $40 million dollars in 2021 in the form of grants for public and private organizations to work together to alleviate healthcare worker shortage in rural areas. The grants are for training and employment programs (https://www.dol.gov/newsroom/releases/eta/eta20210114-0) [Press release].

Fortunately, millennials are choosing to be nurses at a higher rate than baby boomers, and it is projected that the US will only experience shortages in certain geographic areas (Buerhaus et al., 2013). The same holds true for doctors (Fodeman & Factor; 2015). The projected retirements concomitant with physicians' plans to work part-time, further exacerbate this shortage. Again, as with nurses, some geographical areas like the northeast will have a surplus whereas areas like California will have a shortage.

In addition, due to the historical advent of COVID-19, several nurses are considering delaying retirement, partly because of the desire to have more finances when they leave the workforce, and partly because of the need for nurses. Indeed, several nurses came out of retirement to become frontline workers during this pandemic.

Strategies have also been implemented in many states. For example, a nursing student at the University of Wisconsin can receive fellowships and loan forgiveness if s/he agrees to teach in the state after graduation. In Minnesota, clinical sites were expanded through a partnership with the Veteran Administration's healthcare system which allowed for increased enrollment in University of Minnesota's BSN program.

The shortage due to burnout can be mitigated by decreasing the patient: nurse ratio (Chen et al., 2019). This increases nurse job satisfaction and reduces nurse injuries. California has a nurse-to-patient ratio law which is protective for both parties and positively impacts their healthcare organizations. Although there are variations of this strategy, combating the shortage would lead to better nurse-to-patient ratios in every state.

Because PAs can provide many of the same services as physicians, they are expected to continue to have a growing role in providing healthcare services (Hariharan, 2015). This is efficient being that they can be trained more quickly than physicians and can switch to a different area in medicine without investing additional years to be formally trained (Kuriakose, 2020). Although PAs serve different roles than physicians and have not trained as extensively, they are an integral part of the care team and can help mitigate the effects of not having enough doctors to treat patients. Also, as PAs and physicians work together to provide patient care and this approach is continuously developing and expanding to be more efficient (Hackey et al., 2018). Especially as the needs for specialists change depending on the most pressing current threat. For example, an individual with COVID-19 demands a different treatment plan vs. someone suffering from cocaine addiction and a PA can assist with both. Insurance companies are also relaxing their requirements regarding who provides care and now covers physician assistant services. Barriers to growing the number PAs include not having enough clinical sites for the training (Ruopp et al., 2019).

Mental Health Workers

Non-licensed mental healthcare workers with a bachelor's degree in psychology can fill the gap caused by the shortage of licensed mental healthcare professionals. It was shown that similar psychological improvements were achieved regarding patient care (Kunick et al., 2017). This cost-effective model also allows for targeted training in geriatrics while closing disparities experienced by marginalized populations. Emergency medical technicians and paramedics are already used in this manner as they provide care under the supervision of the licensed physicians (Kellerman et al., 2013). Also, although less than 2% of PAs work in psychiatry, recent findings show their ability to treat patients with depression, substance abuse, and other mental health disorders is on par with physicians and psychiatrists (Maudlin et al., 2020).

Improving K12 Science and Math Preparation

As mentioned in the introduction, basic science, and math K12 preparation are instrumental for success in introductory STEM courses. The global ranking of the US in science and math is cause for concern and outreach to K12 teachers and students to enhance continuing education and preparation, respectively. Focusing on building better mathematics and science learning experiences can help alleviate this challenge (Moakler & Kim, 2014). STEM readiness benchmarks for high school or 1st year college freshman students can help stakeholders identify those most likely to succeed in the first-year mathematics and science courses important for STEM success (Chen, 2013). It has been shown that advanced mathematics coursework taken at the high school level leads to better outcomes at the collegiate level (Gayles & Ampaw, 2011). Being that success in mathematics (Cohen and Kelly; 2019) is a strong predictor of persistence in introductory science courses and hence, an indication of a student's likelihood of graduating from a nursing program, it is imperative that high schools enhance their math curriculum.

Higher Education Efforts

Several higher education administrators are implementing strategic action plans to address academic deficits. Math and reading acumen is critical for success in introductory science courses and universities are providing skilled professionals to teach students outside of their classroom instruction. Hence, structural supports like tutoring, supplemental instruction, study hall, *etc.* are in place to help students who did not have access K12 AP math and science courses, or the critical reading skills needed to ensure STEM success in college.

Diversity and Inclusion Efforts

The COVID-19 pandemic caused people from all demographics to witness the impact an inadequate healthcare system has on patient care. Even before the coronavirus began infecting people on a global scale, there was a shortage of diverse nurses, doctors, physician assistants, mental health providers, *etc*. Currently, African Americans make up only 8.5/4.2 percent of physicians/surgeons, respectively, 13.4 percent of registered nurses, and 9.1 percent of nurse practitioners (US Bureau of Labor Statistics [USBLS], 2018; Table 1) and in most healthcare professions, African Americans comprise less than 10%. This is not representative of the US population which is

Stanford cited that Diversity and Inclusion (D&I) must be ingrained within the culture through the mission statement and assessments within the organization, stakeholders from all levels must be included in discussions to implement efforts. These discussions should include successes and failures with similar organizations for the purpose of reflection on strengths and importantly, begin early in engaging communities and schools to ensure that persons from underrepresented groups get early exposure to fields in medicine (Stanford 2020).

Table 1. Demographics of healthcare workers

	% African American	% Hispanic	% Asian
Physicians	8.5	8.8	22.0
Surgeons	4.2	15.6	13.4
Registered Nurses	13.4	7.9	8.7
Nurse Practitioners	9.1	6.3	3.2
Physician Assistants	6.3	7.9	12.3
Mental Health Counselors	9.4	14.0	2.0

THE INVALUABLE ROLE OF HISTORICALLY BLACK COLLEGES AND UNIVERSITIES

Historically Black Colleges and Universities (HBCUs) healthcare programs' missions include addressing the needs of the historically underserved. Hence, not only are they instrumental in diversifying the healthcare workforce, they are also instrumental in training culturally competent individuals who have the compassion needed to serve marginalized populations (Noonan et al, 2013).

HBCUs are known to provide the psychosocial support needed for students to thrive; hence, they matriculate in an environment that is cognizant of their curricular, co-curricular, and emotional needs (Cantey et al., 2011; Esters and Strayhorn 2013; Jones et al., 2020). Professors and other personnel at the institution can provide valuable "othermothering" style support (Flowers, Scott, Riley, & Palmer, 2015) for students whose families and/or friends may not have the tools to build their confidence.

In addition to support, HBCUs are more budget friendly, costing 30% less than their non-HBCU peer institutions. Both factors are important for lower income and/or first-generation students who need more assistance navigating the college experience while paying for the four-six years needed to graduate. Hence, HBCU graduates tend to have less debt when beginning their allied healthcareer.

Unfortunately, there exists only four HBCUs that grant the Doctor of Medicine. These are Meharry Medical College, Howard University College of Medicine, Morehouse School of Medicine, and Charles R. Drew University of Medicine and Science. Notably, Meharry and Howard together produce over 80% of the African American doctors and dentists. Based on their missions (Table 1), it is evident that addressing health disparities and graduating culturally competent doctors is critical.

Due to racism, several Historically Black Medical Schools (HBMSs) were forced to close. If the five medical schools that existed in the early 20th century (Flint Medical College of New Orleans University, Knoxville Medical College, Leonard Medical School of Shaw University, Louisville National Medical College, and the University of West Tennessee College of Medicine and Surgery–Memphis) remained in existence, through extrapolation of existing data, it is calculated that the US would have realized a 29% increase in the number of graduating African-American physicians in 2019 and by now, substantially reduce or even eliminate health disparities (Bennett et al., 2009; Campbell et al., 2020). Even if only two remained open to give six total, the US would have had 63,088 additional African American practicing physicians between 1910 and present day. Hence, the entire nation and the world is suffering from the closure of these HBMSs.

Being that the quality of the healthcare a patient receives is dependent on medical knowledge and cultural competencies, the missions conveyed in Table 1 show that professionals receiving degrees from HBMSs are able to address the challenges faced by those who have been historically disadvantaged. Hence, HBCUs are needed as they are instrumental in graduating clinicians and researchers dedicated to reduce and ultimately close the health disparities gap (Norris et al., 2009; Whitt-Glover 2019).

Twelve per cent and 10.6% of registered nurses and nurse practitioners, respectively, are African American. In 2020, HBCU's with nursing programs were ranked based on reputation, student satisfaction, cost, salary potential using data from IPEDS, College Scorecard, Niche, and U.S. News & World Report. This led to the following top ten (alphabetically ordered):

Table 2. Remaining historically black medical schools

HBMS	Mission
Charles R. Drew University	Social justice and health equity for underserved populations
Howard University	• Improve the health and well-being of individuals • Prepare physicians and other healthcare professionals to serve the underserved. • Educate disadvantaged students for careers in medicine. • Engage in teaching and research activities that address healthcare disparities • Increase the diversity of the health professional and scientific workforce
Meharry Medical College	Advancing health equity
Morehouse School of Medicine	• Improve the health and well-being of individuals and communities • Increase the diversity of the health professional and scientific workforce • Address primary healthcare through programs in education, research, and service Emphasis on people of color and the underserved urban and rural populations in Georgia, the nation, and the world.

- Alcorn State University in Lorman, Mississippi
- Bowie State University in Prince George's County, Maryland
- Florida Agricultural and Mechanical University in Tallahassee, Florida
- Hampton University School of Nursing in Hampton, Virginia
- Howard University in Washington, DC
- North Carolina A&T State University in Greensboro, North Carolina
- North Carolina Central University in Durham, North Carolina
- Southern University and A&M College's College of Nursing and Allied Health in Baton Rouge, Louisiana
- Tuskegee University in Tuskegee, Alabama
- Winston-Salem State University in Winston-Salem, North Carolina

Table 3. HBCU PA programs designed to mitigate healthcare worker shortage

HBCU	Duration (mos.)	Mission
Charles R. Drew University	27	Improve the health of underserved and reduce/ eliminate health disparities
Meharry Medical College	29	Public health policy and advocacy
Morehouse School of Medicine	26	Improve the health of underserved in Georgia
University of Maryland-Eastern Shore	> 26	Community partnerships
Xavier University of Louisiana	28	Improving the healthcare of diverse communities

Increasing financial support to HBCUs to assist with the healthcare shortage is sorely needed. This would allow for the strengthening of structural support such as tutoring to help students who enter college from K12 with inadequate skills to ensure they succeed in introductory STEM courses. Currently, HBCU faculty and/or administrators must submit competitive proposals to acquire external funds and strategically determine how to sustain the program, if funded. It is well known that HBCU faculty have heavy teaching loads, serve on several committees, and invest valuable time in advising/mentoring students who have been historically marginalized and often underserved in K12 (Thompson-Rogers et al., 2018). This makes it challenging to find time to write competitive proposals. In spite of this, faculty at HBCUs win awards to ensure students are successful, but more can be done to increase the funds available so more meritorious awards can be made. Title III funding should be increased to HBCUs to help add more structural support such as tutoring, hiring of more faculty to teach additional sections of STEM and allied health courses, and providing on-campus jobs for students (this leads to higher GPAs). Several schools use Peer-Led Team Learning (PLTL) to foster STEM content mastery (Eren-Sisman, Cigdemoglu, & Geban, 2018; Stephenson, Miller, & Sadler-McKnight, 2019). Title III funds could be used to pay students to tutor in the PLTL program. This would strengthen the foundational knowledge of the peer tutor and help budding healthcare workers excel in their STEM courses. This would also assist students who chose to attend graduate school and receive masters and/or doctoral degrees in healthcare-related professions. Another consequence is the increase in the number of students receiving STEM degrees as they also face the same challenges as allied health majors and would benefit from the same structural support. This is critical because the STEM workforce is also suffering from the lack of diversity and inclusion.

Regarding HBMSs, it is imperative that funds be increased substantially to expand their ability to graduate more doctors. This would assist in diversifying the physician workforce and increase the number of physicians who can help with closing the health disparities gap (Campbell, 2020). Four additional HBCUs should be supported to start a medical school and sustainability funds awarded initially to ensure the new HBMSs obtain accreditation. In addition, the top performing HBCU nursing programs should be given additional funds to expand their programs and avoid turning away qualified applicants.

The HBCUs that are best at graduating mental healthcare workers according to data should also be given funds to increase budgets connected to expanding their programs that will support faculty hires. This would lead to an increase in graduating bachelor, masters, and doctoral level students who earn their rightful place in the healthcare industry (Tucker and Windsor, 2013; Wilbur et al., 2020).

Federal agencies and private corporations fund a plethora of projects and data from these awards can be used to support the allocation of additional funds. Successful pipeline programs that increase the number of students who graduate from healthcare programs should be given additional funds to strengthen their infrastructure and build capacity. For example, postbaccalaureate programs instrumental in diversifying the clinical and especially the physician workforce has proven to be effective and warrant expansion (Arora et al., 2011; Andriole et al., 2015).

Healthcare costs reached $3.8 trillion in 2019 and is expected to increase by at least by 4.6% as in previous years. It is estimated that closing the health disparities gap would save $93 billion/year in medical care costs and $42 billion/year in lost productivity (Turner, 2018). The investment in preparing the next generation of culturally competent healthcare workers who graduate from HBCUs would ultimately lead to an overall higher quality of life for all Americans concomitant with saving taxpayer dollars.

REFERENCES

Alexander, G., Rumay, J. (2021). Disruptive Demographics. *Nursing Administration Quarterly: 45*(1), 58-64 doi:10.1097/NAQ.0000000000000449

Andriole, D. A., McDougle, L., Bardo, H. R., Lipscomb, W. D., Metz, A. M., & Jeffe, D. B. (2015). Postbaccalaureate premedical programs to promote physician-workforce diversity. *Journal of best practices in health professions diversity: research, education and policy, 8*(1), 1036–1048.

Arora, V., Schneider, B., Thal, R., & Meltzer, D. (2011). Design of an Intervention to Promote Entry of Minority Youth into Clinical Research Careers by Aligning Ambition: The TEACH (Training Early Achievers for Careers in Health) Research Program. *The Journal of Social Issues, 67*(3), 580–598. doi:10.1111/j.1540-4560.2011.01715.x

Ayanian, J. Z. (2020). Mental Health Needs of healthcare Workers Providing Frontline COVID-19 Care. *JAMA Health Forum, 1*(4), e200397–e200397. doi:10.1001/jamahealthforum.2020.0397 PMID:36218605

Bennett, K., Philips, J., & Teevan, B. (2009). Closing the Gap: Finding and Encouraging Physicians Who Will Care for the Underserved. *AMA Journal of Ethics, 11*(5), 390–398. doi:10.1001/virtualmentor.2009.11.5.pfor1-0905 PMID:23195179

Bryk, A. S., & Treisman, U. (2010). Make math a gateway, not a gatekeeper. *The Chronicle of Higher Education*, B19–B20.

Buerhaus, P. I., Auerbach, D. I., Staiger, D. O., & Muench, U. (2013). Projections of the long-term growth of the registered nurse workforce: A regional analysis. *Nursing Economics*, *31*(1), 13–17. PMID:23505738

Bureau of Labor Statistics. (2021). *Labor Force Statistics from the Current Population Survey.* [Data set]. U.S. Department of Labor. https://www.bls.gov/cps/cpsaat11.htm (visited *March 09, 2021*).

Campbell, K. M., Corral, I., Infante Linares, J. L., & Tumin, D. (2020). Projected Estimates of African American Medical Graduates of Closed Historically Black Medical Schools. *JAMA Network Open*, *3*(8), e2015220–e2015220. doi:10.1001/jamanetworkopen.2020.15220 PMID:32816033

Cantey, N. I., Bland, R., Mack, L. R., & Joy-Davis, D. (2013). Historically Black Colleges and Universities: Sustaining a Culture of Excellence in the Twenty-First Century. *Journal of African American Studies*, *17*(2), 142–153. doi:10.100712111-011-9191-0

Castro Lopes, S., Guerra-Arias, M., Buchan, J., Pozo-Martin, F., & Nove, A. (2017, March 1). A rapid review of the rate of attrition from the health workforce. *Human Resources for Health*, *15*(1), 21. doi:10.118612960-017-0195-2 PMID:28249619

Cohen, R., & Kelly, A. M. (2020). Mathematics as a factor in community college STEM performance, persistence, and degree attainment. *Journal of Research in Science Teaching*, *57*(2), 279–307. doi:10.1002/tea.21594

Eren-Sisman, E., Cigdemoglu, C., & Geban, O. (2018). The effect of peer-led team learning on undergraduate engineering students' conceptual understanding, state anxiety, and social anxiety. *Chemistry Education Research and Practice*, *19*(3), 694–710. doi:10.1039/C7RP00201G

Esters, L. L., & Strayhorn, T. L. (2013). Demystifying the Contributions of Public Land-Grant Historically Black Colleges and Universities: Voices of HBCU Presidents. *Negro Educational Review*, *64*(1-4), 119–134.

Flowers, A. M., Scott, J. A., Riley, J. R., & Palmer, R. T. (2015). Beyond the call of duty: Building on othermothering for improving outcomes at Historically Black Colleges and Universities. *Journal of African American Males in Education*, *6*(1), 59–73.

Fodeman, J., & Factor, P. (2015). Solutions to the Primary Care Physician Shortage. *The American Journal of Medicine*, *128*(8), 800–801. doi:10.1016/j.amjmed.2015.02.023 PMID:25840033

Gayles, J. G., & Ampaw, F. D. (2011). Gender matters: An examination of differential effects of the college experience on degree attainment in STEM. *New Directions for Institutional Research, 2011*(152), 19–25. doi:10.1002/ir.405

Hackey, R., Grasso, V., LaRochelle, M., Seaver, K. (2018). Rethinking the shortage of primary care physicians, *Journal of the American Academy of Physician Assistants, 31*(6), 47-50 doi:10.1097/01.JAA.0000533662.88073.15

Hariharan, S. (2015). Using Advance Practice Registered Nurses And Physician Assistants To Ease Physician Shortage. *Physician Leadership Journal*, *2*(3), 46–51. PMID:26214952

Holman, E. A., Thompson, R. R., Garfin, D. R., & Silver, R. C. (2020). The unfolding COVID-19 pandemic: A probability-based, nationally representative study of mental health in the United States. *Science Advances*, *6*(42), eabd5390. doi:10.1126ciadv. abd5390 PMID:32948511

Jones, L. V., Ahn, S., Quezada, N. M., & Chakravarty, S. (2020). Enhancing counseling services for Black college women attending HBCUs. *Journal of Ethnic & Cultural Diversity in Social Work*, *29*(4), 325–340. doi:10.1080/15313204.2018.1449689

Juraschek, S. P., Zhang, X., Ranganathan, V. K., & Lin, V. W. (2019). United States Registered Nurse Workforce Report Card and Shortage Forecast. *American Journal of Medical Quality*, *34*(5), 241–249. doi:10.1177/1062860619873217 PMID:31479295

Kandrack, R., Barnes, H., & Martsolf, G. R. (2019). Nurse Practitioner Scope of Practice Regulations and Nurse Practitioner Supply. *Medical Care Research and Review: MCRR*. doi:10.1177/1077558719888424 PMID:31729899

Kandrack, R., Barnes, H., & Martsolf, G. R. (2019). Nurse Practitioner Scope of Practice Regulations and Nurse Practitioner Supply. *Medical Care Research and Review: MCRR*, (November). doi:10.1177/1077558719888424 PMID:31729899

Kellermann, A. L., Saultz, J. W., Mehrotra, A., Jones, S. S., & Dalal, S. (2013). Primary care technicians: A solution to the primary care workforce gap. *Health Affairs*, *32*(11), 1893–1898. doi:10.1377/hlthaff.2013.0481 PMID:24191077

Kichloo, A., Albosta, M., Dettloff, K., Wani, F., El-Amir, Z., Singh, J., Aljadah, M., Chakinala, R. C., Kanugula, A. K., Solanki, S., & Chugh, S. (2020). Telemedicine, the current COVID-19 pandemic and the future: A narrative review and perspectives moving forward in the USA. *Family Medicine and Community Health*, *8*(3), 530. doi:10.1136/fmch-2020-000530 PMID:32816942

Kirch, D. G., & Petelle, K. (2017). Addressing the Physician Shortage: The Peril of Ignoring Demography. *Journal of the American Medical Association*, *317*(19), 1947–1948. doi:10.1001/jama.2017.2714 PMID:28319233

Kunik, M. E., Mills, W. L., Amspoker, A. B., Cully, J. A., Kraus-Schuman, C., Stanley, M., & Wilson, N. L. (2017). Expanding the geriatric mental health workforce through utilization of non-licensed providers. *Aging & Mental Health*, *21*(9), 954–960. doi:10.1080/13607863.2016.1186150 PMID:27243369

Kuriakose, S. (2020, September 11). Pandemics and Mental Health: An Unfortunate Alliance. *SN Comprehensive Clinical Medicine*, *1-5*(11), 2197–2201. doi:10.100742399-020-00501-y PMID:32954209

Kurtzman, E. T., Barnow, B. S., Johnson, J. E., Simmens, S. J., Infeld, D. L., & Mullan, F. (2017). Does the Regulatory Environment Affect Nurse Practitioners' Patterns of Practice or Quality of Care in Health Centers? *Health Services Research*, *52*, 437–458. doi:10.1111/1475-6773.12643 PMID:28127773

Lepkowsky C. M. (2020). Telehealth Reimbursement Allows Access to Mental healthcare During COVID-19. *The American journal of geriatric psychiatry*, *28*(8), 898–899. doi:10.1016/j.jagp.2020.05.008

Mann, D. M., Chen, J., Chunara, R., Testa, P. A., & Nov, O. (2020). COVID-19 transforms healthcare through telemedicine: Evidence from the field. *Journal of the American Medical Informatics Association: JAMIA*, *27*(7), 1132–1135. doi:10.1093/jamia/ocaa072 PMID:32324855

Mauldin, S. G., Morton-Rias, D., Barnhill, G. C., Kozikowski, A., & Hooker, R. S. (2020). The role of PAs in providing mental healthcare. *Journal of the American Academy of PAs*, *33*(12), 34–41. doi:10.1097/01.JAA.0000694988.35913.1a PMID:33234894

Moakler, M. W. Jr, & Kim, M. M. (2014). College Major Choice in STEM: Revisiting Confidence and Demographic Factors. *The Career Development Quarterly*, *62*(2), 128–142. doi:10.1002/j.2161-0045.2014.00075.x

Mossburg, S. E. (2018, March). Baby boomer retirement: Are you up to the challenge? *Nursing Management*, *49*(3), 13–14. doi:10.1097/01.NUMA.0000530428.53528.f2 PMID:29485466

Nguyen, J., Liu, A., McKenney, M., Liu, H., Ang, D., & Elkbuli, A. (2021). Impacts and challenges of the COVID-19 pandemic on emergency medicine physicians in the United States. *The American Journal of Emergency Medicine*, *48*, 38–47. doi:10.1016/j.ajem.2021.03.088 PMID:33836387

Noonan, A., Lindong, I., & Jaitley, V. N. (2013). The role of historically black colleges and universities in training the healthcare workforce. *American Journal of Public Health, 103*(3), 412–415. doi:10.2105/AJPH.2012.300726 PMID:22897530

Norris, K. C., Baker, R. S., Taylor, R., Montgomery-Rice, V., Higginbotham, E. J., Riley, W. J., Maupin, J., Drew-Ivie, S., Reede, J. Y., & Gibbons, G. (2009). Historically Black Medical Schools: Addressing the Minority Health Professional Pipeline and the Public Mission of Care For Vulnerable Populations. *Journal of the National Medical Association, 101*(9), 864–872. doi:10.1016/S0027-9684(15)31032-4 PMID:19806842

Reith, T. P. (2018). *Burnout in United States Healthcare Professionals: A Narrative Review*. Cureus. doi:10.7759/cureus.3681

Ruopp, M. D., Fiore, L., Baughman, A. W., Stern, A. A., Nathan, S. N., & Vilbrun-Bruno, S. (2019). Addressing the Shortage of Physician Assistants in Medicine Clerkship Sites. *Federal practitioner: For the healthcare professionals of the VA. DoD, and PHS, 36*(9), 415–419.

Stanford, F. C. (2020). The Importance of Diversity and Inclusion in the Healthcare Workforce. *Journal of the National Medical Association, 112*(3), 247–249. doi:10.1016/j.jnma.2020.03.014 PMID:32336480

Stephenson, N. S., Miller, I. R., & Sadler-McKnight, N. P. (2019). Impact of peer-led team learning and the science of writing and workshop template on the critical thinking skills of first-year chemistry students. *Journal of Chemical Education, 96*(5), 841–849. doi:10.1021/acs.jchemed.8b00836

Thomas, L. R., Ripp, J. A., & West, C. P. (2018). Charter on Physician Well-being. *Journal of the American Medical Association, 319*(15), 1541–1542. doi:10.1001/jama.2018.1331 PMID:29596592

Thompson-Rogers, K., Davis, D., Davis-Maye, D., & Turner, C. (2018, Summer). Historically Black Colleges and Universities' mentorship of health profession students: A content analysis exploring the North Carolina healthcareers Access Program. *IAFOR Journal of Education, 6*(2), 17–32. doi:10.22492/ije.6.2.02

Tucker, C., & Winsor, D. (2013). Where extrinsic meets intrinsic motivation: An investigation of Black student persistence in pre- healthcareers. *Negro Educational Review, 64*(1–4), 37–57.

Turner, A. (2018). *The Business Case for Racial Equity, A Strategy for Growth.* W.K. Kellogg Foundation and Altarum. https://altarum.org/publications/the-business-case-for-racial-equity-a-strategy-for-growth

Vespa, J., Medina, L., & Armstrong, D. (2020). Demographic turning points for the United States: Population projections for 2020 to 2060. *Current Population Reports. Series P-28, Special Censuses*, 25–1144.

Whitt-Glover, M. (2019). Diversifying the Healthcare Workforce can Mitigate Health Disparities. *Journal of Best Practices in Health Professions Diversity*, *12*(1), III–VI. doi:10.2307/26894222

Wilbur, K., Snyder, C., Essary, A. C., Reddy, S., Will, K. K., & Mary Saxon. (2020). Developing Workforce Diversity in the Health Professions: A Social Justice Perspective. *Health Profession Education*, *6*(2), 222–229. doi:10.1016/j.hpe.2020.01.002

Yates, S. W. (2020). Physician Stress and Burnout. *The American Journal of Medicine*, *133*(2), 160–164. doi:10.1016/j.amjmed.2019.08.034 PMID:31520624

Zhang, X., Lin, D., Pforsich, H., & Lin, V. W. (2020). Physician workforce in the United States of America: Forecasting nationwide shortages. *Human Resources for Health*, *18*(1), 8. doi:10.118612960-020-0448-3 PMID:32029001

Chapter 8
Advocating for Pharmacist Provider Status in the U.S. Healthcare System

Yifei Liu
https://orcid.org/0000-0003-3597-8706
University of Missouri-Kansas City, USA

ABSTRACT

When assessing the needs for a comprehensive national health system, the perspectives toward the current healthcare workforce are necessary. Pharmacists have long been integral professionals in the U.S. healthcare system. They have expanded their scope of practice to increase patients' access to care, improve patients' health outcomes, and reduce healthcare costs. However, they have not been recognized as healthcare providers under the Social Security Act. This chapter aims to advocate for pharmacists' provider status on the federal level. Specifically, there are three learning objectives: 1. To describe the background and efforts for pharmacists to obtain provider status; 2. To demonstrate the benefits of the expanded pharmacy practice scope using two selected pharmacy services; 3. To discuss the future of pharmacy practice.

INTRODUCTION

When assessing the needs for a comprehensive national health system, the perspectives toward the current healthcare workforce are necessary. In the U.S., on one hand, the demand for healthcare products and services has increased; and on the other hand, the shortage of healthcare professionals continues to be an issue. Furthermore,

DOI: 10.4018/978-1-6684-4060-5.ch008

pharmacists have not operated at the top of their licenses, not because of lack of education, training, or clinical skills, but due to exclusion of eligibility as healthcare providers from the Social Security Act.

This chapter aims to advocate for pharmacists' provider status on the federal level. Of note, "provider status" in this chapter refers to federal provider status, and does not include state-level provider status which pharmacists have already achieved in many states. Specifically, there are three main objectives:

1. To describe the background and efforts for pharmacists to obtain provider status;
2. To demonstrate the benefits of the expanded pharmacy practice scope using two selected pharmacy services;
3. To discuss the future of pharmacy practice.

The chapter comprises four sections. The first three sections correspond to the three learning objectives, respectively. The first section describes the context and efforts. The second section focuses on two pharmacy services as examples of expanded pharmacy practice scope, and thus highlights the necessity to support pharmacists' provider status. The third section discusses the future of pharmacy practice, such as further expansion of pharmacy practice scope and advanced roles of pharmacists. The last section provides a summary and concludes that advocacy for pharmacists' provider status is imperative.

BACKGROUND

There is a wide range of healthcare occupations in the U.S. But under Section 1861 (s) (2) of the Social Security Act, only several types of healthcare workers are recognized as providers of medical or other health services by the federal government (U.S. Social Security Administration, 1935). With "provider status", these workers have practice authority and can request reimbursement under Medicare Part B for their healthcare services. Pharmacists have long been integral professionals in the U.S. healthcare system. According to the Bureau of Labor Statistics, the number of pharmacists were 323,500 in 2021 (Bureau of Labor Statistics, U.S. Department of Labor, 2022). In addition, pharmacists are the most accessible healthcare professionals, with almost 90% of Americans reside within 5 miles of a community pharmacy (Berenbrok et al., 2022). Meanwhile, pharmacists have expanded their scope of practice beyond dispensing medications, such as Medication Therapy Management (MTM), immunization, point-of-care testing, smoking cessation, disease state management, transitions of care, and so on. In spite of the easy accessibility within communities and the expanded pharmacy practice to care for patients, pharmacists have not been recognized as providers by the federal government.

The American Pharmacists Association (APhA), the largest association of pharmacists in the U.S., explicitly points out that the top priority of the pharmacy profession is Medicare provider status recognition. APhA states that "Provider status would align reimbursement with the services pharmacists are trained to provide and give underserved patients more access to crucial care" (American Pharmacists Association, 2021). It has issued provider status statements for stakeholders within and outside of pharmacy, including legislative communities and private payers. In addition to APhA, other national pharmacy organizations have also made efforts to achieve pharmacists' provider status. For example, American Society of Health-System Pharmacists, the society representing pharmacists working in hospitals, health systems, ambulatory clinics, and other healthcare settings, has developed an online resource center for Provider Status Readiness (American Society of Health-System Pharmacists, 2022). Furthermore, the Future of Pharmacy Care Coalition, a coalition of pharmacy advocacy organizations for federal policies, has been formed to "recognize and advance the critical role pharmacists play to care for patients and ensure they can continue to create a more just and sustainable healthcare system" (Future of Pharmacy Care Coalition, 2022). The coalition members currently include APhA, American Society of Health-System Pharmacists, AmerisourceBergen, Cardinal Health, CVS Health, Good Neighbor Pharmacy, Health Mart, Kroger, Medicine Shoppe, McKesson, National Association of Chain Drug Stores, and Walgreens.

Despite the efforts made by national pharmacy organizations, to achieve provider status, legislations would need to happen on the federal level. Therefore, actions from the Congress, the legislative branch consisting of the House of Representatives and the Senate, would be vital. So far, the Pharmacy and Medically Underserved Areas Enhancement Act, has been introduced to the Congress to amend the Social Security Act by including pharmacists as healthcare providers. For the 114th Congress (2015-2016), it was introduced to the House of Representatives as H.R.592 and to the Senate as S.314 (H.R. 592, 2015-2016; S.314, 2015-2016). For the 115th Congress (2017-2018), it was introduced to the House of Representatives as H.R.592 and to the Senate as S.109 (H.R. 592, 2017-2018; S.109, 2017-2018). For the 117th Congress (2021-2022), it was introduced to the House of Representatives as H.R. 2759 and to the Senate as S.1362 (H.R. 2759, 2021-2022; S.1362, 2021-2022). The bill gathered bipartisan support in the 114th Congress (2015-2016) and the 115th Congress (2017-2018), but the progress ended with the phase of being introduced to the House of Representatives and the Senate. If it became law, the bill would allow pharmacists to provide certain already-authorized services in a medically underserved area or for a medically underserved population, and receive reimbursement for these services from Medicare Part B. Medically underserved area is a geographic area that has a shortage of primary care health services, and medically underserved population is a population subset that has such a shortage within a geographic area (Health Resources and Services Administration, U.S. Department of Health and Human Services, 2022).

For the 117th Congress (2021-2022), the Equitable Community Access to Pharmacist Services Act, was also introduced to the House of Representatives as H.R.7213 (H.R. 7213, 2021-2022). The context of this bill is the increasing demand for healthcare services in under-represented, underserved, and rural communities owing to coronavirus disease 2019 (COVID-19). Pharmacists have worked on the front lines to combat the pandemic, as more than 291.5 million doses COVID-19 vaccines have been administered at community pharmacies (U.S. Centers for Disease Control and Prevention, 2022). If it became law, the bill would allow pharmacists to receive reimbursement under Medicare B for testing and administering vaccines for COVID-19 and influenza, testing for respiratory syncytial virus and strep throat, and the initiation of drug regimens to treat COVID-19, influenza, or strep throat (H.R. 7213, 2021-2022). The legislation efforts are supported by the Future of Pharmacy Care Coalition along with over 100 companies, associations, and organizations (Future of Pharmacy Care Coalition, 2022).

As mentioned earlier, both the Pharmacy and Medically Underserved Areas Enhancement Act, as well as the Equitable Community Access to Pharmacist Services Act are currently in the phase of being introduced to the 117th Congress (2021-2022). The former was introduced to both the House of Representatives and the Senate, and it is not a new bill. The latter is a new bill which was introduced to the House of Representatives only. The next phase for either bill would be the passage in the House of Representatives or the Senate by the conclusion of the 117th Congress on January 3, 2023. However, the prospect of either bill moving to the next phase is unclear. When the Pharmacy and Medically Underserved Areas Enhancement Act was introduced to the 114th Congress (2015-2016), a concern over its fate was the budgetary implications due to the compensation for pharmacists under Medicare Part B (Harper, 2015). At present, the same budgetary implications would still stand, and the House of Representatives or the Senate would weigh the benefits versus the expenses if either bill is chosen to move forward. Nevertheless, it is up to pharmacists to educate the public, other healthcare professionals, third party payers, policymakers, and legislators about the benefits of obtaining provider status for patient care, and garner support or sponsorship for these legislation efforts.

EXPANSION OF PHARMACY PRACTICE SCOPE

Expanding the scope of pharmacy practice is not the same as achieving provider status, as pharmacists can expand their scope of practice without provider status. Yet, without provider status, the bottleneck to expand pharmacists' scope of practice is the lack of a federal reimbursement mechanism like Medicare Part B. Many private payers also use the mechanism of Medicare Part B to design their coverage. The expansion of pharmacy practice scope would not be sustainable in the long run, and pharmacists' access to provide already-authorized services would be limited. This is because pharmacists would not be able to consistently receive reimbursement for these services from government or private payers. The sustainability issue would further cause suboptimal care for patients as patients would not be able to benefit from these pharmacy services.

Pharmacists have offered a variety of pharmacy services notably distinct from dispensing medications. This section does not have space to detail every pharmacy service mentioned in the first section. Rather, it focuses on Medication Therapy Management (MTM) and immunization as two examples to illustrate the benefits of pharmacy services and the necessity to keep them available to patients.

Medication Therapy Management (MTM)

MTM originates from the Medicare Prescription Drug, Improvement, and Modernization Act of 2003 which established Medicare Part D and included MTM as a paid service under Medicare Part D (Public Law 108-173, 2003). After the bill became law, 11 national pharmacy organizations developed a consensus definition of MTM as (Bluml, 2005):

"Medication Therapy Management is a distinct service or group of services that optimize therapeutic outcomes for individual patients.

Medication Therapy Management services are independent of, but can occur in conjunction with, the provision of a medication product.

Medication Therapy Management encompasses a broad range of professional activities and responsibilities within the licensed pharmacist's, or other qualified healthcare provider's, scope of practice. These services include but are not limited to the following, according to the individual needs of the patient:

a. Performing or obtaining necessary assessments of the patient's health status

b. Formulating a medication treatment plan

c. *Selecting, initiating, modifying, or administering medication therapy*
d. *Monitoring and evaluating the patient's response to therapy, including safety and effectiveness*
e. *Performing a comprehensive medication review to identify, resolve, and prevent medication-related problems, including adverse drug events*
f. *Documenting the care delivered and communicating essential information to the patient's other primary care providers*
g. *Providing verbal education and training designed to enhance patient understanding and appropriate use of his/her medications*
h. *Providing information, support services, and resources designed to enhance patient adherence with his/her therapeutic regimens*
i. *Coordinating and integrating medication therapy management services within the broader healthcare management services being provided to the patient*".

Generally speaking, pharmacists can manage prescription medications in MTM, as patients progress through their medication therapies. Pharmacists can prevent adverse effects, identify medication-related problems, customize medication treatment plans to patient needs, and provide valuable feedback to prescribers and patients regarding treatment outcomes including adherence. Interestingly, medication-related problems identified and resolved were the two most common outcome measures among MTM studies (Viswanathan et al., 2014). According to a systematic review and meta-analysis of 44 MTM studies, MTM has improved medication appropriateness, adherence, and percentage of adherent patients, and reduced medication dosing (Viswanathan et al., 2015). Although evidence is insufficient to evaluate the effectiveness of MTM on most outcome measures (Viswanathan et al., 2015), improved medication appropriateness and adherence, as well as reduced dosing are likely to lower overall healthcare expenditures. The cost savings would not only come from improved medication utilization, but also from reduced utilization of unnecessary emergency room visits or hospitalization. For instance, in an employer-sponsored MTM program for diabetic patients, a total cost savings of $179,047.80 was made after considering the costs of emergency room visits, inpatient visits, and visits to a physician' office (Pinto et al., 2013). A quasi-experimental study of 2,083 older adults reported an MTM program of "Pharm2Pharm" reduced medication-related hospitalization by 36% and realized a 2.6:1 return on investment (Pellegrin et al., 2017).

In 2021, the spending on prescription drugs in the U.S. reached to $576.9 billion, with a growth rate of 7.7% from 2020 (Tichy et al., 2022). Adalimumab, a specialty medication, was the top drug by overall expenditure of $28.5 billion (Tichy et al., 2022). Specialty medications are often injectable biologics to treat complex conditions (Academy of Managed Care Pharmacy, 2019). Compared with traditional medications, specialty medications cost more, and may require expertise in administration and intense monitoring. In 2021, the spending on specialty medications totaled $284.9 billion, nearly half of the prescription drugs expenditures, with a growth rate of 8.7% from 2020 (Tichy et al., 2022). The rising costs of prescription drugs including specialty medications, has placed MTM of particular importance to support the management of specialty medications. The Academy of Managed Care Pharmacy comments that pharmacists who handles specialty medications should "have the capability to administer prior authorization programs to ensure appropriate use and capture the necessary data for ongoing monitoring", as well as "work closely with physicians and case managers to ensure medication adherence, resolve any problems and coordinate changes in therapy" (Academy of Managed Care Pharmacy, 2019).

Immunization

In the U.S., the Advisory Committee on Immunization Practices (ACIP) develops vaccine recommendations and guidelines, and the Centers for Disease Control and Prevention determines the immunization schedules for children and adults (Advisory Committee on Immunization Practices (ACIP), U.S. Centers for Disease Control and Prevention, 2013; U.S. Centers for Disease Control and Prevention, 2022). As of July 5, 2022, the Food and Drug Administration (FDA) lists 104 vaccines licensed for use in the U.S. (U.S. Food and Drug Administration, 2022). However, there are unmet immunization needs among adults. For example, although ACIP recommends that all adults aged 50 and over to receive two doses of shingles vaccine, only 34.5% of adults aged 60 and over received a shingles vaccine in 2018 (Dooling et al., 2018; Terlizzi & Black, 2020).

Pharmacists are essential healthcare professionals to meet the immunization needs of the public. They have been involved in immunization programs with various roles across various healthcare settings. One example is their hard work to administer COVID-19 vaccines, which was mentioned earlier in the context of the Equitable Community Access to Pharmacist Services Act. Another example is Project VACCINATE, a one-year demonstration project in 70 community pharmacies in Washington State (Bacci et al., 2019). The project resulted in a 15% increase in the total number of vaccines administered, including influenza, pneumococcal, pertussis, and herpes zoster vaccines. Pharmacists can administer vaccines in every state, but their immunization authority varies by state in terms of types of vaccines and whether a prescription is needed (American Pharmacists Association and National Alliance of State Pharmacy Associations, 2022). APhA has developed the following guidelines for pharmacy-based immunization advocacy and administration (American Pharmacists Association, 2019):

"Guideline 1 – Prevention – Pharmacists should protect their patients' health by being vaccine advocates.

Guideline 2 – Partnership – Pharmacists will be a member of the immunization neighborhood by collaborating, coordinating, and communicating with immunization stakeholders to protect the community from vaccine-preventable diseases.

Guideline 3 – Quality – Pharmacists must achieve and maintain competence to administer immunizations.

Guideline 4 – Documentation – Pharmacists should document immunizations fully and report clinically significant events appropriately.

Guideline 5 – Empowerment – Pharmacists should educate patients about immunizations and respect patients' rights."

A systematic review and meta-analysis of 36 studies examined the impact of pharmacists on immunization rates (Isenor et al., 2016). Despite the roles of pharmacists in immunization programs (whether they were educators, facilitators, or administrators of vaccines) or the types of vaccines, pharmacists' involvement led to increased immunization rates. Another systematic review and meta-analysis analyzed 8 studies in which pharmacists were the administers of vaccines, and also revealed significant positive impact on immunization rates (Baroy et al., 2016).

FUTURE OF PHARMACY PRACTICE

This section discusses the future of pharmacy practice from two viewpoints – further expansion of pharmacy practice scope and advanced roles of pharmacists. Provider status would promote further expansion of pharmacy practice scope by the same rationale described in the previous section. Again, using MTM as an example, the U.S. Centers for Medicare and Medicaid Services tested an Enhanced MTM model from 2017 to 2022 (U.S. Centers for Medicare and Medicaid Services, 2022). Compared with the traditional MTM model, the features of the Enhanced MTM model include more payment incentives and regulatory flexibilities, and the expected outcomes include improved quality of care and reduced net Medicare expenditures.

Using pharmacists' endeavors to combat COVID-19 as another example, the Test-to-Treat COVID-19 Initiative was launched in March 2022 (U.S. Administration for Strategic Preparedness and Response, 2022). A person can get tested for COVID-19, and the test is positive and a treatment is appropriate, the person can receive a prescription and have it filled at one location. The Test-and-Treat locations include pharmacy-based clinics, federally-funded health centers, long-term care facilities, community-based sites, and federally-supported Test-to-Treat sites (U.S. Administration for Strategic Preparedness and Response, 2022). Additionally, in July 2022, the FDA authorized pharmacists to prescribe Paxlovid to eligible patients with certain limitations (U.S. Food and Drug Administration, 2022). The director of the FDA's Center for Drug Evaluation and Research stated the reason as "Since Paxlovid must be taken within five days after symptoms begin, authorizing state-licensed pharmacists to prescribe Paxlovid could expand access to timely treatment for some patients who are eligible to receive this drug for the treatment of COVID-19" (U.S. Food and Drug Administration, 2022).

For the pharmacist workforce, designations of advanced practice pharmacists have emerged in four states - advanced practice pharmacist in California, clinical pharmacist practitioner in Montana and North Carolina, and pharmacist clinician in New Mexico (Frost & Adams, 2018). For example, to become an advanced practice pharmacist in California, in addition to holding an active pharmacist license, a candidate must meet two of three criteria: being a board certified pharmacy specialist, completing a residency, or providing clinical services for at least one year under a collaborative practice agreement (California State Board of Pharmacy, 2022). There has not been not much uptake for advanced practice pharmacist designations (Frost & Adams, 2018). In addition, it is hard to tell how provider status could impact these designations. If pharmacists' provider status was recognized, some pharmacists might be interested in obtaining the designations to perform more responsibilities, whereas others might not be interested as some responsibilities associated with the designations could be performed with provider status.

Collaborative working relationships with other healthcare professionals could facilitate pharmacists to expand their scope of practice, or carry out responsibilities under the designations of advanced practice pharmacists. Unfortunately, the American Medical Association (AMA) is against pharmacists' expanding roles in providing COVID-19 vaccines to children aged between 3 and 18, in the Test-to-Treat Initiative, under H.R.7213, and prescribing Paxlovid (American Medical Association, 2020; American Medical Association, 2022a; American Medical Association, 2022b; Madara, 2022). APhA firmly opposes to AMA's current stance (American Pharmacists Association, 2022a; American Pharmacists Association, 2022b). In addition, executives of APhA and the National Community Pharmacists Association rejected AMA's objection on pharmacists' prescriptive authority of Paxlovid (Blank, 2022). Regardless of AMA's opinions, administering COVID-19 vaccines for children aged 3 and above, conducting Test-to-Treat Initiative, and prescribing Paxlovid become available at community pharmacy locations. For example, Walgreens started administration of COVID-19 vaccines to children 3 years old and above at select locations nationwide (Walgreen Co, 2022). Furthermore, an APhA report stresses that the expanded pharmacy practice scope has been complementary to physicians' practice, and supports collaborative patient care models with physicians (Liu, 2022).

CONCLUSIONS

In the U.S., pharmacists have expanded their scope of practice to increase patients' access to care, improve patients' health outcomes, and reduce healthcare costs. However, they have not been recognized as healthcare providers under the Social Security Act, so they are not able to receive reimbursement for their services from Medicare Part B. The lack of reimbursement affects the sustainability of their services and the optimal care for patients. To achieve provider status for pharmacists would require legislations to happen on the federal level. Currently, two bills to amend the Social Security Act to include pharmacists' provider status, the Pharmacy and Medically Underserved Areas Enhancement Act, and the Equitable Community Access to Pharmacist Services Act, are in the phase of being introduced to the 117th Congress (2021-2022). Obtaining provider status would not only release pharmacists' full potential to provide care but also benefit patients. In addition, pharmacists' scope of practice will continue to evolve, and provider status would promote further expansion of pharmacy practice. Pharmacists need to educate the public, other healthcare professionals, third party payers, policymakers, and legislators about why obtaining provider status is imperative.

REFERENCES

Academy of Managed Care Pharmacy. (2019). *Specialty Pharmaceuticals, Concepts in Managed Care Pharmacy, Managed Care Pharmacy 101*. Available at: www.amcp.org/about/managed-care-pharmacy-101/concepts-managed-care-pharmacy/specialty-pharmaceuticals

Advisory Committee on Immunization Practices (ACIP), U.S. Centers for Disease Control and Prevention. (n.d.). *ACIP Vaccine Recommendations and Guidelines*. Available at: https://www.cdc.gov/vaccines/hcp/acip-recs/index.html

American Medical Association. (2020). *AMA opposes expanding pharmacists' ability to provide child vaccines*. Press release. Available at: www.ama-assn.org/press-center/press-releases/ama-opposes-expanding-pharmacists-ability-provide-child-vaccines

American Medical Association. (2022a). *AMA statement on Administration's test-to-treat COVID-19 plan.* Press release. Available at: www.ama-assn.org/press-center/press-releases/ama-statement-administration-s-test-treat-covid-19-plan

American Medical Association. (2022b). AMA statement on Paxlovid prescribing. Press release. Available at: www.ama-assn.org/press-center/press-releases/ama-statement-paxlovid-prescribing

American Pharmacists Association. (2022a). *APhA House of Delegates passes policy addressing access to pharmacist-provided services*. Available at: www.pharmacist.com/Pharmacy-News/apha-house-of-delegates-passes-policy-addressing-access-to-pharmacist-provided-services

American Pharmacists Association. (2022b). *APhA addresses AMA's inaccurate description of H.R. 7213 and viewpoints of most physicians working alongside pharmacists*. Press release. Available at: www.pharmacist.com/APhA-Press-Releases/apha-addresses-amas-inaccurate-description-of-hr-7213-and-viewpoints-of-most-physicians-working-alongside-pharmacists

American Pharmacists Association. (2021). *Pharmacy's Top Priority: Medicare Provider Status Recognition.* Available at: www.pharmacist.com/Advocacy/Issues/Medicare-Provider-Status-Recognition

American Pharmacists Association. (2019). *Guidelines for Pharmacy-based Immunization Advocacy and Administration*. Available at: aphanet.pharmacist.com/sites/default/files/files/Guidelines_for_Pharmacy_Based_IMZ_Advocacy_Approved_Jan_26_2019.pdf

American Pharmacists Association and National Alliance of State Pharmacy Associations. (2022). *Pharmacist administered vaccines*. Available at: www.pharmacist.com/DNNGlobalStorageRedirector.ashx?egsfid=EACvwV2aS-8%3d

American Society of Health-System Pharmacists. (2022). *Provider Status Readiness*. Available at: www.ashp.org/pharmacy-practice/resource-centers/provider-status-readiness

Bacci, J. L., Hansen, R., Ree, C., Reynolds, M. J., Stergachis, A., & Odegard, P. S. (2019). The effects of vaccination forecasts and value-based payment on adult immunizations by community pharmacists. *Vaccine*, *37*(1), 152–159. doi:10.1016/j.vaccine.2018.11.018 PMID:30446177

Baroy, J., Chung, D., Frisch, R., Apgar, D., & Slack, M. K. (2016). The impact of pharmacist immunization programs on adult immunization rates: A systematic review and meta-analysis. *Journal of the American Pharmaceutical Association*, *56*(4), 418–426. doi:10.1016/j.japh.2016.03.006 PMID:27450138

Berenbrok, L. A., Tang, S., Gabriel, N., Guo, J., Sharareh, N., Patel, N., Dickson, S., & Hernandez, I. (2022). Access to community pharmacies: A nationwide geographic information systems cross-sectional analysis. *Journal of the American Pharmacists Association*, *62*(6), 1816–1822.e2. Advance online publication. doi:10.1016/j.japh.2022.07.003 PMID:35965233

Blank, C. (2022). *Pharmacy groups respond to AMA criticism on pharmacists prescribing Paxlovid*. Available at: www.drugtopics.com/view/pharmacy-groups-respond-to-ama-criticism-on-pharmacists-prescribing-paxlovid

Bluml, B. M. (2005). Definition of medication therapy management: Development of professionwide consensus. *Journal of the American Pharmaceutical Association*, *45*(5), 566–572. doi:10.1331/1544345055001274 PMID:16295641

Bureau of Labor Statistics, U.S. Department of Labor. (2022). *Occupational Outlook Handbook, Pharmacists*. Available at: www.bls.gov/ooh/healthcare/pharmacists.htm

California State Board of Pharmacy. (2022). *Advanced Practice Pharmacist information*. Available at: www.pharmacy.ca.gov/applicants/app.shtml

Dooling, K. L., Guo, A., Patel, M., Lee, G. M., Moore, K., Belongia, E. A., & Harpaz, R. (2018). Recommendations of the Advisory Committee on Immunization Practices for use of herpes zoster vaccines. *MMWR. Morbidity and Mortality Weekly Report*, *67*(3), 103–108. doi:10.15585/mmwr.mm6703a5 PMID:29370152

Frost, T. P., & Adams, A. J. (2018). Are advanced practice pharmacist designations really advanced? *Research in Social & Administrative Pharmacy*, *14*(5), 501–504. doi:10.1016/j.sapharm.2017.10.002 PMID:29097045

Future of Pharmacy Care Coalition. (2022). Available at: pharmacycare.org/support/

Harper, P. C. (2015). Pharmacist provider status legislation: Projections and prospects. *Journal of the American Pharmaceutical Association*, *55*(2), 203–207. doi:10.1331/JAPhA.2015.14176 PMID:25749265

Health Resources and Services Administration, U.S. Department of Health and Human Services. (2022). *What is Shortage Designation?* Available at: bhw.hrsa.gov/workforce-shortage-areas/shortage-designation

H.R. 2759 - Pharmacy and Medically Underserved Areas Enhancement Act, 117th Congress (2021-2022). Available at: www.congress.gov/bill/117th-congress/house-bill/2759

H.R. 592 - Pharmacy and Medically Underserved Areas Enhancement Act, 114th Congress (2015-2016). Available at: www.congress.gov/bill/114th-congress/house-bill/592

H.R. 592 - Pharmacy and Medically Underserved Areas Enhancement Act, 115th Congress (2017-2018). Available at: www.congress.gov/bill/115th-congress/house-bill/592

H.R. 7213 - Equitable Community Access to Pharmacist Services Act, 117th Congress (2021-2022). Available at: www.congress.gov/bill/117th-congress/house-bill/7213

Isenor, J. E., Edwards, N. T., Alia, T. A., Slayter, K. L., MacDougall, D. M., McNeil, S. A., & Bowles, S. K. (2016). Impact of pharmacists as immunizers on vaccination rates: A systematic review and meta-analysis. *Vaccine*, *34*(47), 5708–5723. doi:10.1016/j.vaccine.2016.08.085 PMID:27765379

Liu, Y. (2022). Passion and purpose drive the 2022 APhA House of Delegates sessions. APhA–APRS, The potential impact on science and research. *Journal of the American Pharmaceutical Association*, *62*(4), 918–919. doi:10.1016/j.japh.2022.05.023

Madara, J. (2022). *Letter to Representatives Kind and McKinley*. Available at: searchltf.ama-assn.org/letter/documentDownload?uri=%2Funstructured%2Fbinary%2Fletter%2FLETTERS%2F2022-4-12-Letter-to-Kind-and-McKinley-re-HR-7213-Equitable-Community-Access-to-Pharmacists-v3.pdf

Pellegrin, K. L., Krenk, L., Oakes, S. J., Ciarleglio, A., Lynn, J., McInnis, T., Bairos, A. W., Gomez, L., McCrary, M. B., Hanlon, A. L., & Miyamura, J. (2017). Reductions in medication-related hospitalizations in older adults with medication management by hospital and community pharmacists: A quasi-experimental study. *Journal of the American Geriatrics Society*, *65*(1), 212–219. doi:10.1111/jgs.14518 PMID:27714762

Pinto, S. L., Kumar, J., Partha, G., & Bechtol, R. A. (2013). Improving the economic and humanistic outcomes for diabetic patients: Making a case for employer-sponsored medication therapy management. *ClinicoEconomics and Outcomes Research*, *5*, 153–159. PMID:23610526

Public Law 108-173, Medicare Prescription Drug, Improvement, and Modernization Act of 2003, 108th Congress (2003-2004). Available at: www.govinfo.gov/app/details/PLAW-108publ173

S.109 - Pharmacy and Medically Underserved Areas Enhancement Act, 115th Congress (2017-2018). Available at: www.congress.gov/bill/115th-congress/senate-bill/109

S.1362 - Pharmacy and Medically Underserved Areas Enhancement Act, 117th Congress (2021-2022). Available at: www.congress.gov/bill/117th-congress/senate-bill/1362

S.314 - Pharmacy and Medically Underserved Areas Enhancement Act, 114th Congress (2015-2016). Available at: www.congress.gov/bill/114th-congress/senate-bill/314

Terlizzi, E. P., & Black, L. I. (2020). *Shingles vaccination among adults aged 60 and over: United States, 2018. NCHS Data Brief, no 370*. National Center for Health Statistics.

Tichy, E. M., Hoffman, J. M., Suda, K. J., Rim, M. H., Tadrous, M., Cuellar, S., Clark, J. S., Ward, J., & Schumock, G. T. (2022). National trends in prescription drug expenditures and projections for 2022. *American Journal of Health-System Pharmacy*, *79*(14), 1158–1172. doi:10.1093/ajhp/zxac102 PMID:35385103

U.S. Administration for Strategic Preparedness and Response. (n.d.). *Test to Treat*. Available at: aspr.hhs.gov/TestToTreat/Pages/default.aspx

U.S. Centers for Disease Control and Prevention. (2022). *The federal retail pharmacy program for COVID-19 vaccination*. Available at: www.cdc.gov/vaccines/covid-19/retail-pharmacy-program/index.html

U.S. Centers for Disease Control and Prevention. (2013). *Immunization Schedules*. Available at: www.cdc.gov/vaccines/schedules

U.S. Centers for Medicare and Medicaid Services. (n.d.). *Part D Enhanced Medication Therapy Management Model*. Available at: innovation.cms.gov/innovation-models/enhancedmtm

U.S. Food and Drug Administration. (2022). *Vaccines licensed for use in the United States*. Available at: www.fda.gov/vaccines-blood-biologics/vaccines/vaccines-licensed-use-united-states

U.S. Food and Drug Administration. (2022). *Coronavirus (COVID-19) update: FDA authorizes pharmacists to prescribe Paxlovid with certain limitations*. Available at: www.fda.gov/news-events/press-announcements/coronavirus-covid-19-update-fda-authorizes-pharmacists-prescribe-paxlovid-certain-limitations

U.S. Social Security Administration. Compilation of the Social Security Laws, Sec. 1935. [42 U.S.C. 1395x]. Available at: www.ssa.gov/OP_Home/ssact/title18/1861.htm

Viswanathan, M., Kahwati, L. C., Golin, C. E., Blalock, S., Coker-Schwimmer, E., Posey, R., & Lohr, K. N. (2014). *Medication Therapy Management Interventions in Outpatient Settings. Agency for Healthcare Research and Quality (US).* Available at: www.ncbi.nlm.nih.gov/books/NBK294478

Viswanathan, M., Kahwati, L. C., Golin, C. E., Blalock, S. J., Coker-Schwimmer, E., Posey, R., & Lohr, K. N. (2015). Medication therapy management interventions in outpatient settings: A systematic review and meta-analysis. *JAMA Internal Medicine*, *175*(1), 76–87. doi:10.1001/jamainternmed.2014.5841 PMID:25401788

Walgreen Co. (2022). *Walgreens now providing Pfizer and Moderna COVID-19 vaccines to children ages 3 and older at select locations nationwide*. Available at: news.walgreens.com/press-center/news/walgreens-now-providing-pfizer-and-moderna-covid-19-vaccines-to-children-ages-3-and-older-at-select-locations-nationwide.htm

Section 3
Cultural and Institutional Attributes

Chapter 9
Untold Stories:
Healthcare, Education, and Social Justice for African Americans

Darryl Scriven
Clarkson University, USA

ABSTRACT

African Americans have been impacted by lack of access to quality health care as well as affordable health care for over 100 years in the United States. One of the most horrifying and public consequences of this was the U.S. Department of Public Health's Study of Untreated Syphilis in the African American Male conducted in rural Macon County, Alabama from 1933 to 1973. It is stories like this, when told, that have the power to impact institutional research board policies and institute standards like "informed consent" to protect human subjects. In this chapter, the author recounts three narratives as a heuristic device to personalize the modern health care history of African Americans, as well as argue for what can be done to ameliorate health care disparities and prevent excess black deaths.

INTRODUCTION

All communities tell stories. In fact, communities are often defined by who understands the stories being told as well as how and why those stories have shared meaning. Our stories weave a tapestry of nourishing connection from our individual experiences to affirm and preserve our "Us-ness". As the African proverb goes, "I AM" *because* "WE ARE". But "WE ARE" because our stories perform purposeful, unifying, and sometimes unrecognized Sankofa rituals in our lives. No matter how

DOI: 10.4018/978-1-6684-4060-5.ch009

edifying or brutal they may be, the telling of our stories gathers a people together to transmit information, identity, and strength for the journey. And wherever you find yourself, the stories on which you were nursed will largely determine how you live, with whom you identify, and ultimately who you think you are.

Yet, when our stories are untold, we wander about failing to decipher codes cracked by our ancestors long ago. When our stories are untold we fail exams, not because we lack knowledge but because we lack an interconnected perspective of the oneness of all things. When our stories are untold, we feel alone like suffering Souls on Ice rather than feeling part of a shared consciousness rooted in creativity, collective work, and responsibility. When our stories are untold, we act against our own interests. We act against our children. We act against ourselves. And we are doomed to repeat the same cycles until our stories awaken our whole existence, from time immemorial until now.

As we Commemorate this 25th Anniversary of the Presidential & National Apology for the United States Department of Public Health's Study of Untreated Syphilis in the African American Male, the task today is simple: as an exemplar of transparency, this chapter candidly unpacks and lays bare three stories. These stories will demonstrate how education, healing, and social justice are necessary ingredients of a 3-sided pyramid. But the stories will also demonstrate that, without the unifying foundation of neighbor love, deep education, true healing, and abiding social justice can never be achieved. While portraying individual experiences, like the Syphilis Study, these stories are profoundly universal in that they reflect our shared aspiration, suffering, striving, and inevitable triumph. Also like the Syphilis Study, these stories have African Americans in the Deep South and health insurance at the center. Our first protagonist is Mary Scriven, the second is Samuel Scriven, and the third is Johnathan Story.

MARY SCRIVEN

Mary Alice Scriven, my mother, was born to the union of Mary Jane and Leotis Scriven on December 25, 1944 in Jacksonville, Florida. She had two sisters and a brother, but Mary was the youngest. Due to her youth, she remained at home when the other siblings either came of age to start families or moved away for college. Mary finished high school in the early 1960's and sought vocational training as a Medical Assistant. Since both her parents would soon after be diagnosed with cancer, her training and familiarity with the healthcare system would prove to be an asset. Still, quality affordable healthcare in the 1960's and early 1970's was difficult for everyday people to access, particularly for working class African Americans who did not have health insurance through their jobs. It's hard being sick and poor at the same time, because poverty compounds sickness in a society where healthcare is for sale and sold high above the poverty line.

Enter me in December 1973. My grandmother had passed on before I was born, and my grandfather 2 years after I was born. My mother was unmarried but inherited the family home so we had a place to live with some ancestral memory. All of this occurred at a time before legal safeguards for working mothers were firmly in place but at a time when President Nixon, masterminded by Pat Buchanan, vetoed federal daycare legislation that would have enabled me to attend free preschool during the day while my mother worked. Nevertheless, my mother was able to continue her employment as a Medical Assistant. Also, fortunately for us, my grandfather's sister, Aunt Sweets, came from Pittsburgh to live with us. This prevented her from going to a nursing home and eased the burden of single parenting on us (which is how family works). Despite Nixon and Buchanan's argument that free daycare would turn poor kids into Chinese Red Communists, my mother paid for me to go to preschool and we all benefitted from her employer-sponsored healthcare.

Enter my sister Kimberly in February 1979. My Aunt Sweets has moved to an Independent Living Community and my mother's employer has relocated to a section of town that is inaccessible without a car at 7:30 in the morning, given small children and a single-parenting situation. With this loss of employment and health insurance –facing minimum-wage alternatives that would not cover the cost of daycare– my mother reluctantly decided to apply for public assistance and Medicaid, allowing her to stay home with us until my sister was school age.

So, my mother worked that plan as best she could in the midst of Trickle-down Reaganomics and the hyperbolic, degrading, and scapegoating imagery of Cadillac Welfare Queens, but we soon found that there was sometimes a different caliber of regard and treatment given to Medicaid patients than to those with non-governmental health plans. Services covered under Medicaid might not always be suggested to patients by providers because the state reimbursements were often lower than the plan payments. Or patients on Medicaid might encounter a hostile treatment environment as if they were stealing services they were unentitled to instead of justly receiving benefits they had paid for many times over. Worse still, when I would be brought in with sprains or sports injuries, my mother being eyed with suspicion as if the default paradigm was to presume child abuse, or at least neglect, about poor black parents on Medicaid. Given enough of these episodes between seeking healthcare for me and my sister (because my mother rarely, if ever, sought care for herself), the unspoken household rule became "only go to the doctor if the pain is unbearable". I agree with Warren and Katz that the data do not suggest that African Americans inordinately avoid treatment due to mistrust of the healthcare providers *per se*, yet more work needs to be done to ascertain the impact of dignity assaults on deterring patients, especially black, brown, poor, and female patients, from pursuing primary care, specialty care, and mental health services.

Before re-entering the workforce, my mother trained to be both a dental assistant and nursing assistant so she could access jobs closer to our home. In fact, I never sat in a dentist's chair until I was 21-years old because my mother would regularly remove calculus from my gum line with a hand tool and monitor my teeth for cavities before school. And while she was glad to be working for an African American Dentist in walking distance from home, the new job paid minimum wage with no health benefits. But for personal and generational dignity, she worked 6 out of 7 days for $180 a week. This was not a salary. This was a $4 hourly wage that amounted to less than $10,000 a year, and we had no health insurance. We were considered part of the Working Poor; people who worked all day but still lived below the poverty line without insurance or a safety net.

Taking sick days meant a dip in weekly pay; so, there were no sick days. Thus, in addition to dignity assaults as Medicaid patients, my mother's wage-punitive work schedule without insurance benefits was a second barrier to us accessing healthcare. I would watch my mother wrap her swollen ankles in ace bandages and walk to work. She would stand on her feet all day, walk home, and literally fall asleep in her work clothes before making dinner. But then she started to suffer from daily headaches. To self-medicate, she would send me to the corner store to get an RC Cola and packet of BC or Goody powder. At the same time, she told me and my sister, "I do this so you won't have to" and "If you keep believing, keep working hard, and do your best in school, life will get better". So, all my sister and I knew to do was to keep believing, keep working hard, and to do our best in school. It paid off.

Taking cues from my mother and my community, I applied to Florida A&M University (FAMU). At FAMU, I received a full scholarship that covered tuition, fees, room, board, $1,000 a semester and, if I chose a public Florida University, a fellowship that covered to the end of my Ph.D. A profound yet easily overlooked benefit of my student status was being covered by student health insurance. During my first two years at FAMU, I held a 4.0 GPA and it seemed that troubles were a thing of the past. But in April of my sophomore year, I received a call from my 12-year old sister. She said, "Mom lost the peripheral vision in her right eye 3 days ago but kept going to work and never told her boss because she was afraid she'd lose her job. And she didn't want me to call you because she knew you were taking your finals." Thankfully, I had finished my last final and was able to buy our first family car by saving my educational stipend money, so I raced home as fast as I could. By the time I reached Jacksonville, again because of my sister, mom had been taken to the Emergency Room by a church member. Unfortunately, she had a debilitating stroke the next day.

We learned that her constant headaches were symptoms of many small strokes over the years and now, at 47, years of being untreated had manifested.[1] So, mom spent a month in the hospital and a month in rehabilitation. I couldn't think about returning to school because I had to take care of my mother. Another well-meaning church member told me, "Your mother wouldn't want you to drop out of school, so why don't you put her in a nursing home?" My response was that, "My mother wouldn't put me in a nursing home. I'm not putting her in a nursing home." Instead, I packed up the house and moved mom and my sister to Tallahassee with me and we lived in an apartment off of that scholarship money and I finished my undergraduate degrees 2 years later. The education that my mother worked so diligently for us to have literally took care of us; and my mother's sacrifice, while not unique, was a heavy sacrifice that allowed our family to have 16 more years of life together and, for that reason alone, was not in vain.

SAMUEL SCRIVEN

Samuel Scriven, our son, was born in Baton Rouge, Louisiana on October 25, 2002. He is the third child and only son of a father born in Jacksonville, Florida and a mother born in the Tabasco capitol of the world –New Iberia, Louisiana. We named him specifically after that biblical prophet because they sensed he would be a special child with a deep connection to life and people, making a contribution that would move humanity forward in some way. All parents may desire this for their children but Samuel's parents independently *understood it*. We *felt* it; like my Aunt Sweets could tell that it was going to rain when there were no clouds in the sky –because she *felt it* in her joints.

As University Professors, health insurance was a feature of our employment, and seeking care for ourselves and our children was no longer a concern I had. According to Samuel's ultrasound images, he was progressing nicely in the womb and would arrive right on schedule. But when Samuel was born, it was discovered that he had a tiny hole in his heart. The physician said that Samuel could have an irregular heartbeat but that the hole should close over time on its own. I was born with a hole in my heart that had closed on its own, so we were fairly confident that Samuel's heart would be fine. A more immediate concern were Samuel's feet and ankles. When Samuel was born, instead of his feet and legs being perpendicular, the tops of his feet were touching the outer sides of his shins. Seeking out a specialist, as young parents, we were told that if Samuel ever walked, he would walk with his feet at almost a 180 degree angle.

Latricia and I have no medical training. My wife grew up in a family of teachers and I grew up working poor. We had no illusions about relying on political parties to help people. Our parents taught us that *people* help people and it is often the case that people help those with whom they share a common bond or experience –a story. And when our stories overlap and intersect, our motivation to help each other is stronger. Even though my and Latricia's origins were radically different, the common strands that knit our shared story together were Intentional Education and Applied Faith.

All of our parents taught us that Education was an essential key to both enjoying and protecting ourselves from a world that had much to offer, but would sometimes seek to harm us for being brilliant while black. So in an epoch of open access and Affirmative Action, they intentionally steered us toward Historically Black Colleges and Universities for our foundation –to connect our head and our hands to our hearts, our minds to our meaning, and our purpose to our people. Thus, when we met at Purdue University for graduate study, we knew that the only way to survive was for us to protect each other from those who would resist the image our parents had imprinted on our souls.

With that in mind, Latricia heard what the physician said about Samuel's feet, but his words didn't match the image that she had of our son in her heart. We respected his medical training, but our intentional education had taught us how to find information for ourselves and how to come to our own conclusions before the advent of Google and YouTube. Sam was given orthopedic casts to wear and he wore them daily. But Latricia, through diligent research and Applied Faith, believed that if she prayed and rotated our son's ankles several times a day in addition to him wearing the casts, that his ankle bones were malleable enough to be reformed in the way they should go. So she did that. And in 3-months time, when we returned to the specialist for a check-up, he could not believe that Samuel's feet were straight and his ankles were strong and at normal angles.

Beyond being a pianist, guitarist, thespian, and All-State Chorus member, our son Samuel was MVP each of the 7 years he played basketball and now does gymnastics on his way to high school. The medical opinion given could have been understood by us as an insurmountable fact of life. It was instead treated as an informed, yet alterable, perspective on our son's future. As Latricia rotated his ankles, when our son cried, she cried too –matching our son's sacrifice and healing us all in the process. Her intentional education from a Historically Black Southern University complemented her self-image with credentialed competency; this combined with her love and mother-wit enabled her to be a peer in the midst of power. Still, it would be a gross oversight to ignore the griot role of quality health insurance in my son's narrative.

In an environment where privilege is normal, it could be easy to miss all of the puddles that quality health insurance equips one to sidestep. Yet, being connected to an ongoing narrative informs us that healing is an outgrowth of love, environment, and resources. To understand my son's story is to understand that my mother's story is one ancestral groan of people who knew that intentional education was not only social alchemy but a spiritual pursuit that would transform global probabilities and allow humanity to become radical by definition–actually seeing the root of the matter.

JOHNATHAN STORY

Johnathan Story is the root of the matter. Johnathan was born in Atlanta, Georgia on December 27, 1986. He attended and played football at Maryville College in Tennessee. As a student-athlete, Johnathan had his share of minor football injuries but enjoyed the coverage of team health insurance that left him with no worries. Everyone on the team and afterwards called him Story, so I will refer to him in the same way here. Once he graduated, Story came back to Atlanta, got a job, and lived at home with his mother Lurene and his 16-year old sister Jessica. I met Story at church in 2013 and noticed that he was a big guy with a friendly disposition and had a beautiful singing voice. He was 26 at the time and a member of the young adult ministry at St. James United Methodist Church in Alpharetta, GA. I saw him at church on Sundays and we shared humorous exchanges somedays after service.

In October of that year, one of the couples at the church hosted their baby shower at our home. Many in the young adult ministry attended, including Story, and we had a really good time. During the event, someone heard our son, Samuel, shooting hoops in the driveway and, as young men tend to do, a group of guys started playing basketball. At that point, my son was 10 years old and had the agility of a cat. So, when Story went out to guard him, Sam crossover dribbled like an NBA hopeful, went to the basket, and brought the ball back after finishing the shot. Meanwhile, Story had fallen to the ground and the other guys were having a hearty laugh about him getting schooled by an elementary student. But Story stayed on the ground clutching his knee and everyone knew that the injury was serious.

My son ran in crying and told me he felt responsible for what had happened. I reassured him that it wasn't his fault and, when I went outside, I could see that Story's kneecap was turned sideways on his leg. We told Story he should go to the hospital but his reply through gritted teeth was, "I can't go. I don't have insurance." After writhing in pain for another 45 minutes, he finally allowed us to lift him up and place him in a car to go to the Emergency Room where he could receive treatment with or without insurance. Story had a job, but the health insurance offered by his employer was cost-prohibitive and he deemed it too big of an expense because he provided much of the household income for his mother and sister. Three of the guys went with him to the Emergency Room, so I stayed to console my son and attend to the guests inside who had no idea of the severity of what had just occurred.

When Story arrived at the hospital, he learned that he needed surgery to correct his dislocated kneecap. Yet, instead of operating on him then or the next day, the attending physician and hospital sent him home that Saturday night with some crutches, a prescription for pain killers, and a surgery date of Monday. *Monday*. No time for the surgery was given, but Story was told that he would receive a phone call with instructions the next day. Sunday came and went, no phone call. Monday came and went, no phone call. His close buddies said he remained in good spirits but felt that he had been sent home and overlooked because he didn't have health insurance. Story felt "put on the back burner" because his pain wasn't as lucrative as insured pain. He did finally receive a call on Tuesday and was told that his surgery had been rescheduled to Friday.

However, on Wednesday he called to tell his mother that he wasn't feeling well. During the conversation, his mother says that he abruptly stopped responding. She frantically called his name and rushed home to find him lifeless on the floor. The autopsy revealed that her son had died from an aneurism caused by a blood clot that traveled from his knee to his brain. Professor Cornel West rightly admonishes us that one necessary condition of truth is to allow suffering to speak. Story's suffering was the kind of preventable, senseless, unnecessary, excess death without dignity that terrorized the uninsured daily because of the way our society was structured. Story's death occurred two months before the Affordable Care Act mandate took effect and that legislation would have given him more empowerment in his treatment decision and would almost certainly have saved his life.

HEALING AND INSURANCE

I have written elsewhere about the Affordable Care Act and how it, even more than President Clinton's heartfelt sentiments or the establishment of the Tuskegee University National Center in Bioethics in Research and Healthcare, represents a robust apology and distributive justice for the USPH Syphilis Study (Scriven, 2015). It is no mystery that the seducing element in 1932 Macon County was the US Public Health Department's promise of "free" treatment in a context where the target population lacked access to health insurance and affordable healthcare. I wrote in the aforementioned piece that, "President Obama's Affordable Care Act is the social policy that turns words into justice, for Tuskegee and for the American people as a whole. While the men of Macon County provided the context, the promise of the

Clinton Apology was essentially to secure justice for all people exposed to health disparities exacerbated by low income, lack of insurance coverage, lack of access, and a price insensitive healthcare market. Obamacare is the United States making good on that National Promise; realized when all the six survivors who heard President Clinton's Apology were dead and gone" (Scriven, 2015).

And now the Affordable Care Act is under attack by people who seem to be consciously disconnected from the historical narrative of national integrity and atonement that it represents for crimes against the Souls of Black Folk and sacred humanity alike. In the garb of politicians and economists, they choose to politicize and commodify the lives of the most vulnerable among us. This is why we are here today, to tell the continuing story of our people's enduring struggle for justice and freedom in a context where goods are unjustly distributed. And because we have struggled and lived and care-given and been poor and been ashamed and been exalted and been intentionally educated and been embraced by those who loved us fiercely and taught us the ancestral narrative and fundamental root of the matter. When my 10-year old son, sobbing with his head bowed said to me, "Dad, I feel like I killed Story" –I could look at him in the eyes and imprint on his soul these words. I replied to my son, "Baby, you didn't kill Story. A healthcare system that sent him home without treatment because he didn't have insurance killed Story."

Mary Scriven, Samuel Scriven, and Johnathan Story, all embodying stages along life's way, illustrate how the presence or lack of affordable, quality medical treatment influences the resolution of any narrative. This is why we must intentionally educate ourselves and our children to fight for Healthcare for all people; because its attainment is a triumphant contribution of OUR STORY to humanity. When suffering is truly allowed to speak, then healing and justice can begin.

POSTSCRIPT

While musing these narratives, I realized that most people do not doubt that the U.S. Healthcare System is in need of revision. But what exactly does that mean? Does it mean we need Universal Healthcare? Does it mean that the current system does not treat people fairly? That it is too expensive for the average American to secure medical care? That the system should cover all Americans? That what we have now (Medicare & Medicaid) takes up too much of the national budget for too little return? Or that insurance companies are literally ripping people's eyes out of the sockets by overcharging, refusing payment, dropping coverage, or denying coverage in the interest of pure profit? Again, what exactly do we mean by stating "in need of revision" so we can be clear?

There are all sorts of things that democratically elected governments compel citizens to pay for in the interest of the Republic. Things like roads, schools, fire departments, and police precincts are few examples. Most people accept that these items are in service to the common good and accept the price tag that goes along with them. Still, there are some who insist on fighting each of these in the name of resisting taxation. I presume if I didn't ever drive down Main Street, I could make a case that the portion of my taxes devoted to maintaining Main Street was unjust because I never drive that way. Or that I never call the police, fire department, or don't send my kids to public schools –so those taxes on me are unfair, too. But this argument really misunderstands the idea of the social contract that undergirds the fabric of any society.[2]

To be specific, there was a time when people simply existed by their wits, all alone; them against the world. If a group of bandits rode up to your cabin and demanded all your food, you either gave them the food, fought them off, or died trying. Obviously, if the game was continuously set up this way, the stronger group would consistently win. This would ratify a version of the idiom "Might Makes Right". So, people who didn't want to work their whole lives only to have their possessions stolen or family murdered on the whim of aggressors entered into agreements or contracts called societies. In these societies, individuals come together with the understanding that they are acting in their best personal interest by acting in the best interest of the collective or group. Does that mean that every decision the group makes will sit well with the individual? Of course, not. But the individual is clear on a couple of things. One is that it is better to be a member of a society who is sometimes disgruntled about the group's decisions, than to be out there all alone with no bonds of allegiance strong enough to resist forceful takings. Another is that he or she 'voluntarily' surrenders some of liberty to participate in the social contract and be a part of the Republic. We cannot eat our cake yet, still have it whole on the table. Likewise, it is a misunderstanding of the societal project altogether to suppose that we can have absolute, unrestrained liberty that worships rugged individualism and intentionally tries to share healthcare resources but expects to benefit from a society where people are healthy, content, civil, and optimistic about our future as a nation.

Now what does this have to do with "Universal Healthcare"? I argue that basic, regular healthcare should be accessible to all residents in advanced modern societies. I'm not comfortable with saying the healthcare is a human right or an inalienable right, because this suggests that it should always exist regardless of the circumstances. I don't think that. But the circumstances of America are that we have a mismanaged healthcare system that is in the hands of insurers and medical providers who are making maximum profits at the expense of quality and affordable healthcare. There is nothing wrong with making lots of money. But there is something wrong with tying the profit motive to negative well-being and loss of human life through denial of legitimate health insurance claims. Healthcare professionals are caught in the middle with exorbitant costs/debt, on one hand, and the feeling of entitlement to enormous incomes, on the other. In a country where things can be restructured so that people have access to basic medical care, they should. Anything valuable costs money.

Why is 17% of the US Gross National Product (GNP) spent on healthcare? It is not because of the number of people covered by Medicare & Medicaid. To use a phrase coined by Attorney Timothy Carter, that's what the 'pathological oppositionist' rhetoric would have us think. Instead, the real reason for the high GNP expenditure is price gouging that is a standard practice throughout the healthcare industry. Kenneth Arrow, a 1972 Nobel Prize winning economist, observed that prices are irregularly determined in the healthcare market as opposed to other markets. In a 1963 article published in the *American Economic Review*, Arrow argued that the supply of medical services does not simply depend on the desire of patients, but it is mainly determined by the professional judgment of the physicians –who just happen to be the main economic beneficiaries of the recommended treatment (Arrow, 1963).

As a narrative, let's imagine that a patient comes to see me with partially blocked arteries and describing occasional light-headedness. After examination, I determine that the condition is reversible with medicine, diet, and exercise, but could be immediately treated with plaque removal surgery. I have outstanding student loan bills, and the surgery would definitely bring me the most financial return. Talk about incentives! So, what do I do? Is there any wonder why, over the last twenty years, open-heart surgery has become one of the most common surgical procedures performed in the United States? The average listed price for this procedure is $30,500 (AHA, 2011).[3] It should come as no surprise that physicians are the most influential factors when it comes to treatment choices (Arrow, 1963). Given equally effective treatments, am I going to consistently choose to put people like Patient B on a diet and a treadmill or am I going to lean toward scheduled surgeries? The fact that it's a 'no-brainer' is the problem.

In his book, *A Second Opinion: Rescuing America's Healthcare*, Arnold Relman (2007) agrees with Arrow that "medical services are largely price insensitive." Relman, a former editor-in-chief of the *New England Journal of Medicine* and member of the White House Health Professionals Review Group, underscores my point here. Who's going to shop around for bargain brain surgeries or bid on Craig's List for the cheapest heart surgeon prices when in medical crisis? The truth is that patients have very little bargaining power when their condition is more urgent; and the healthcare system knows it. I am not demonizing doctors or singling-out healthcare providers. But I am emphasizing the phrase Relman (1980) coined in his 1980 *New England Journal of Medicine* article that hyper-commercialization of American medicine constituted a "new medical industrial complex." I am also asserting that the true issue is not insurance, but prices. To remedy this, the national investment should be in medical education to reduce the cost and student loan debt for physicians to attend medical school as well as additional training to expand who can perform medical functions currently relegated to physicians (i.e., physician assistants, nurse practitioners, and nurses).

Such an expansion of training for medical professionals will increase the supply of providers of mundane medical services that do not require all the expertise at a physician's disposal. This increased supply in providers will warrant a justified reduction in prices and lend itself to cost-standardization of certain elements in the medical encounter. There will still be the ability for cost variance due to differentiation, but the public would benefit economically from price-standardization of common services and procedures. As this occurs, demand will inevitably increase and precipitate the need for more medical providers (both domestically and abroad) to be trained and brought into the U.S. Healthcare System. It will be a realignment of the medical profession toward service that makes a good living. To those with means, there will always be concierge medicine to provide a more catered experience. Access is not the enemy of quality. Access is a foundational ingredient of quality. Every business should make money. But it is not congruent with publically expressed American values and evolving standards of global decency to maximize medical profit at the cost of human lives. I have no doubt that my mother, my friend Story, and many in the African American community who have experienced excess death would still be alive today had our healthcare ecosystem been structured around access and prevention instead of exclusivity and price insensitivity.

REFERENCES

AHA. (2011). *Heart Disease and Stroke Statistics* [Data set]. American Heart Association.

Arrow, K. (1963). Uncertainty and the Welfare Economics of Medical Care. *The American Economic Review*, *3*(5), 941–973. https://www.jstor.org/stable/1812044

Hobbes, T. (1651). *Leviathan or The Matter, Forme and Power of a Commonwealth Ecclesiasticall and Civil*. Academic Press.

Relman, A. (1980). The New Medical-Industrial Complex. *The New England Journal of Medicine*, 303.

Relman, A. (2007). *A Second Opition: Rescuing American's Health Care*. Public Affairs.

Scriven, D. (2015). Tuskegee & Obamacare: Fulfilling America's Promise of Health Care Justice. Journal of Healthcare, Science, and the Humanities, 5(2), 113-123.

ENDNOTES

1 At the time of completing this manuscript, I am 47 years of age.

2 See Thomas Hobbes (1651).

3 https://health.costhelper.com/heart-surgery.html#extres1. Accessed March 13, 2021. Also see the 2011 American Heart Association Report, https://www.ahajournals.org/doi/pdf/10.1161/cir.0b013e3182009701. Accessed March 13, 2021.

Chapter 10
Australia's Medicare System:
Learning From Other's Examples

Melissa Robin Bowman Foster
Winston-Salem State University, USA

ABSTRACT

The current United States health care system is continuously falling short of the promises made by numerous political health care leaders. Although some efforts have been made to improve the system, such as the Patient Protection and Affordable Care Act, the current system still leaves a large percentage of the population uninsured or underinsured. Additionally, patients delay seeking care because of the high out-of-pocket costs, which allows conditions to become more severe, therefore leading to more costly treatment and adding to the large amount of money that must be written off by health care organizations. In this chapter, a review is provided of Australia's effort to improve these conditions for Australians through Australia's Medicare program. The chapter will also suggest how some components of the Australian Medicare System could help improve the quality of the United States health care system.

INTRODUCTION

Learning from Others

There are many different types of learning. Observational learning, also known as modeling, is a common style that was first officially labeled by a psychologist, Albert Bandura, in 1986. Observational learning involves the functions of observing the actions of others, retaining what was observed, and then replicating the actions

DOI: 10.4018/978-1-6684-4060-5.ch010

that resulted in positive consequences and avoiding those actions that had negative consequences (Fryling, Johnston, & Hayes, 2011). Observational learning can be seen in many different scenarios by individuals of all ages and by groups representing many different areas. Newborn babies learn their basic steps of communication and human emotion through observational learning. Professional sports teams learn the best maneuvers and tactics to use on their upcoming opponents by observing previous games/matches. It is important to emphasize that observational learning does not simply result in copying the behaviors and/or actions one sees, but rather understands the resulting outcomes of those actions and, based on those, determines if those outcomes are desirable. If so, then the observational learners would then need to apply the observed actions to their own scenarios which may require some modifications pending the similarities and differences between those observers and the observed. Preferably, observers would choose to observe those who have similar qualities so the resulting actions would be as close as possible to what would happen if they were to apply similar processes.

With 195 other countries, the United States has a plethora of potential candidates to observe and review to determine best practices for improving its current healthcare system. Being a developed, democratic country, it would be best to find a country or countries to observe that share these qualities. Since universal healthcare is a topic and potential future that has been discussed for decades in the United States, it would also be preferable to find a country that has similar qualities, offers universal healthcare, and has been successful in this endeavor.

Knowing this, it would be extremely strategic for the United States to look at other developed countries that offer universal healthcare and learn from their methods. Australia is also labeled a developed country. The country's government is made up of three elements: the Parliament which includes the Queen (represented by the Governor-General), the Senate, and the House of Representatives. The structure of Australia's government labels it as a constitutional monarchy and parliamentary democracy. Australia also offers universal healthcare for all citizens and has also earned a reputation for having top quality services as well as a much lower national debt when compared to the United States. When surveying Australian citizens, most express approval and content with their universal healthcare system. Because of these qualities, Australia is a good example to look to when determining steps to take to improve the healthcare system in the United States.

Brief Background of United States' (US) Healthcare System

The United States healthcare system does not currently offer a universal health insurance plan. Although there are some government-sponsored plans offered to limited, qualifying members (Medicare, Medicaid, Tricare, CHAMPVA) of the population, the majority of the population still depends on private insurance.

Strengths of US Healthcare System

Although not perfect, the United States healthcare system does have positive aspects that must be acknowledged. When compared to other countries, access to quality healthcare services in the U.S. is much more rapid. The United State's dependence on private insurance companies contributes to this strength. If a U.S. citizen has quality, private insurance coverage this can ensure ready access to most necessary healthcare services including specialty care and pharmaceuticals because providers know some reimbursement is guaranteed through that patient's private insurance plan (Bhaduri, 2020).

Another aspect to consider is, thanks to a quality higher education system that is constantly growing, there is an ongoing supply of trained medical staff to serve in hospitals and clinics across the country. Although there are always shortages in certain specialty areas –compared to many other countries– the patient to provider ratio is much more desirable. Additionally, thanks to ongoing funding for research and the rapid advances in medical technology, the American healthcare system has provided improved healthcare quality and health status for a large portion of the population. This includes more comfortable medical environments. more sanitary conditions, and the ability to offer patient privacy in treatment areas (Bhaduri, 2020).

For those employed by large companies, employer-sponsored insurance has also ensured a more cost affordable way for citizens to acquire private insurance coverage by providing this coverage to the insured for a discounted, group rate and in some cases the employer will also cover some of the cost (Bhaduri, 2020).

The patient-centered initiative that has been implemented in the U.S. healthcare industry has also improved healthcare quality. The initiative encourages patient empowerment and informed involvement in their own health decisions. Although it may be the normal practice in the U.S. to, as a patient, have a right to choose who you see for medical care as well as the type of treatment you agree to receive, this is not the case in all countries. By having a system that includes "in-network" and "out-of-network" providers listed within a patient's insurance plan, this gives the patient the option to stay with an in-network provider for better financial coverage or, if desired, to pay more out of pocket but receive care from an out-of-network provider (Fix et al., 2018).

Since the implementation of the Patient Protection and Affordable Care Act (PPACA), preventive medicine has also received a long overdue focus and those services are now covered in a much larger aspect than in previous years (Atkinson & Giovanis, 2015).

Weaknesses of US Healthcare System

To improve a system, it is imperative to be aware of and understand the weaknesses of the system.

The first weakness to be acknowledged in the United States' healthcare system is the large percentage of the American population who are uninsured. Approximately 10% of the United States population is uninsured. When the uninsured accrue large medical debt, these unpaid services contribute to the already large debt the healthcare industry is dealing with. Not only is the healthcare industry having to deal with unpaid services from those who are uninsured, there is also a large portion of the population who are underinsured or have inadequate healthcare coverage. Although these citizens may be able to pay for apt of their services, the lack of adequate coverage to ensure payment for the expensive medical costs in the U.S. healthcare system leads to more unpaid debt within the industry. As usual, healthcare costs continue to be the largest spending category in the United States' gross domestic product (GDP), and when compared to other developed countries, the percentage is always much higher. Although the Patient Protection and Affordable Care Act attempted to greatly decrease and ultimately eliminate the number of uninsured, it did not provide much assistance for those who were underinsured but instead, in some ways, contributed to this problem. Although a person may have insurance, he/she will have just as big of a negative impact on the economy and the health of their neighbors if he/she cannot afford to seek preventative care, treatment, and/or pay for the medical services provided.

A second weaknesses closely tied to the first is the expense of healthcare services and products. When reviewing many types of medical procedures, the same procedures of equal or better quality can be received in other countries for a much cheaper price. One of the main causes for this is the lack of central control of inflation of medical costs. Many other countries have central agencies that closely monitor the rates associated with medical services and costs, as well as pharmaceutical and durable medical equipment (DME) costs. With no central controlling agency, and the unique characteristics associated with healthcare marketing and supply and demand, healthcare costs in the United States have been on an erratic and constant increase for decades.

Another weakness is the major gaps in communication. Although somewhat improved since the introduction of computers in healthcare, there are still major gaps when delivering patient information from one provider to another as well as to insurance companies. Patients are constantly undergoing unnecessary procedures due to a lack of communication from one provider to another. For example, oncology patients usually have a large panel of providers due to the necessity of different specialists to monitor their disease progress and treatment. Throughout the patient's care, all of these providers will require blood work to monitor the body systems associated with their specialty. If communicating properly, all necessary tests can be completed during one blood draw, one specimen run, and one patient visit. Unfortunately, due to the lack of communication, patients are constantly having to provide blood samples multiple times within a week (or sometimes day) because one provider did not communicate his/her desired labs to another, and two separate orders come in at different times. Not only does this waste medical supplies due to multiple sticks, it also wastes time and equipment wear and tear due to multiple samples being run on the same patient. And most importantly, the patient is having to be exposed to numerous needle sticks and/or catheter access point sticks and trips to the medical office with an already compromised immune system. Unnecessary patient sticks and office visits increase the chances of nosocomial infections (hospital or medical facility acquired infections) leading the patient to require infection treatment that could have been avoided if the patient had not been required to return for more testing. Scenarios like this are happening daily throughout our country because of lack of communication among providers and leading to the unnecessary use of equipment, supplies, and unnecessary hardships for patients.

Furthermore, if medical providers were communicating adequately with insurance companies, the insurance representatives could also serve as a "check in" point to ensure patients are not having unnecessary, repeated procedures.

Brief Background of Australia's Healthcare System

All Australian citizens are eligible for the country's universal health insurance plan, Medicare. Additionally, when seeking care from public hospitals and certain healthcare providers, patients can receive much of their care with little or no out-of-pocket cost except for prescriptions and some supplementary or specialty services.

Australia's Medicare system is mainly supported by a 2% tax on personal taxable income with low-income citizens being exempt. Australia's Medicare is controlled by all three levels of the government (federal, state/territory, and local). The public hospitals are supported by the states/territories and/or local governments where they are located. The federal government regulates other health services/facilities. The majority of emergency care provided in Australia is at public hospitals. Additionally, Australian citizens have the option to buy into the private health system. Private coverage allows people to seek care at private hospitals and to have additional coverage that is not offered by Australia's Medicare, such as dental and vision. For those in lower income brackets, private coverage can also be purchased and the government will offer a rebate. About half of the Australian population purchases additional private coverage, mainly those with higher incomes. The government does strongly encourage those in higher income brackets to purchase private insurance by requiring them to pay a tax if they don't. Additionally, if a citizen in the higher tax bracket does not purchase coverage before the age of 30, they are at risk of being forced to pay higher premiums (Dixit, 2018).

Strengths of Australia's Healthcare System

One of the main strengths that Australia's healthcare system has over the United States' healthcare system is that there is an option for healthcare coverage available to all Australian citizens. This prevents individuals from accumulating high healthcare costs due to being uninsured and/or underinsured.

The three levels of the government (federal, state/territory, local) communicate very well in regards to national crisis response, medical research funding, veterans care funding, distribution of pharmaceuticals and durable medical equipment, and quality control. This has helped ensure the healthcare services provided are of good quality when compared to many other countries.

Although the government does fund healthcare, they do not provide care and instead leave the quality of care to be determined by medical professionals. This has helped Australia become a country well known for top-quality medical care.

Approximately half of the population still purchase private insurance to assist with coverage gaps in Medicare (dental, vision, etc.) which is subsidized by the government. This subsidization encourages citizens to purchase extra coverage which also ensures adequate reimbursement for services and helps counteract a large, nationwide healthcare debt (Dixit, 2018).

Weaknesses of Australia's Healthcare System

Seeking healthcare from a private hospital is extremely difficult for those who cannot afford private insurance or the self-pay option. Preferably, there would be a way to make private hospitals an option for all citizens regardless of income. Additionally, although the Australian government does limit physicians on how much they can be reimbursed for services, there is no regulations preventing physicians from charging patients more than the allotted amount to make up for any reduction in the amount the government allots for services. Unfortunately, this has led citizens to believe the physicians charging the most also offer better quality services, which is not necessarily true, therefore leading to unnecessary high medical costs and inaccuracies in marketing competition.

Another weakness of Australia's Medicare is failure to provide dental, vision, and long-term care coverage. Citizens are required to seek this coverage from the private sector, which again can be difficult for those in the lower income bracket. This leads to a high number of citizens being underinsured or uninsured in these specific areas.

A third weakness is the lack of coordination of care and other communication within the clinical setting. Australia is controlled by all three sectors of the Australian government – federal, state/territory, and local. The three sectors do demonstrate quality communication regarding items such as, quality control of public healthcare facilities, funding of research, funding of veteran's care, regulation of pharmaceutical devices, responses to national emergencies, and nationwide equitable distribution of healthcare providers. However, gaps in communication have been found at the clinical level when it comes to coordinating care between facilities controlled by different entities. This can delay patient care and ultimately decrease the quality of services provided.

A fourth weakness is shortage of medical professionals. Although the three tiers of government do communicate to ensure equitable distribution of healthcare providers, the problem remains that there is still an overall shortage of healthcare workers throughout the country (Robinson, et al., 2015).

Applying Components of Both Systems for An Improved US Healthcare System

To look at potential improvements of the United States' healthcare system, we will review the previously mentioned weaknesses and apply what we know of Australia's Medicare system to come up with recommended guidance and/or solutions.

The first weakness mentioned was the large percentage of uninsured and underinsured citizens in the United States population. Obviously, providing universal healthcare to all United States' citizens would greatly decrease the amount of care provided to people without insurance. However, to address the additional problem of the large percentage of underinsured citizens, the coverage must be adequate. When reviewing Australia's Medicare system, the areas lacking coverage included vision, dental, and long-term care. As discussed, Australian citizens address these coverage gaps by purchasing additional, supplemental coverage. This system works well, and it also creates and supports an industry which can provide more jobs to citizens (private insurance sector). However, as we can see with the United States, without any major incentives and/or encouragement from the government to urge citizens to purchase private insurance, this will not happen and we will, once again, end up with a large number of uninsured. Again, this is where the United States can look to Australia's practices of requiring citizens within a certain tax bracket to purchase additional, private insurance or otherwise pay a levy.

Similar to the levy required by Australia for citizens who do not purchase additional insurance, the United States initiated a practice with the Patient Protection and Affordable Care Act by charging citizens a penalty if they could not provide proof of insurance coverage for the entire year. Unfortunately, many citizens discovered that insurance is so expensive in the United States that the cheaper option was to pay the penalty. To ensure this practice, or similar ones, will be more successful in the future the government will have to take a more controlling position when it comes to the cost of healthcare insurance as well as services. This will be discussed in more detail further in the chapter.

Additionally, Australia offers set premiums for those who purchase coverage before a certain age. One of the hardships encountered by older citizens is higher premiums for coverage because of the higher risk associated with caring for the elderly. To encourage citizens to seek medical care and coverage early, and to maintain good preventative healthcare practices, Australia will "lock in" citizens to a premium so they cannot be charged a higher amount as they age. To be locked in to the amount, a citizen must purchase coverage before a certain age and maintain that coverage. This program was initiated by Australia in 2000 and called Lifetime Health Cover. The government provides a list of approved health insurance plans for citizens to purchase and maintain in order to be locked in to their premium amount. It is well known that the two main contributing factors for the increase in healthcare costs in the United States are medical advances and the aging population. People are living longer lives thanks to advances in medicine. However, this also means a larger "older" population that will require medical care. Knowing this, and to make it more affordable for U.S. citizens to care for themselves as they age, it is recommended that the United States also consider options for the aging population to ensure a locked in premium for different types of healthcare insurance coverage.

To provide universal healthcare, the United States government will have to find a way to fund the service. This will ultimately lead to an increase in taxes, which will undoubtedly create backlash from the population. It is imperative that the United States communicate how this will ultimately ensure that the average citizen will spend less on their medical care as well as what benefits it will provide to the overall good while improving the nation's debt. The government will need to determine the average amount spent by citizens on healthcare at different life stages. Considering this, the government will need to aim to draw an amount out of individual taxes that will be substantially less than what that citizen would have spent, on average, on his/her own paying for premiums and uncovered expenses. The same must be considered for families and those filing jointly. By coming up with a system that will ultimately ensure individuals are spending less on medical care, while still receiving quality care from desired providers, the government will be able to address and ultimately lessen the criticisms expressed by citizens who are concerned over the increase in taxes. Furthermore, providing forecasts on the impact this will have on the nation's debt as well as the large percentage of the GDP spent on healthcare expenditures, will hopefully assist in easing the concerns many citizens will have.

Again, to make a new universal healthcare system work, the entire cost scheme will have to be reviewed and controlled, which requires to address the second weakness mentioned: the high costs of healthcare services and products. When compared to other countries, healthcare costs in the United States are much higher but do not necessarily produce a better product or service to justify the increased cost. This can be attributed to many factors but one is little to no control over pricing. Pharmaceutical companies are constantly price gouging for medications and/or products that are necessary for a patient's survival and/or quality of life. Physicians and other care providers have responded by doing the same thing when it comes to setting prices for their own services. Australia, although not in the same medical debt as the United States, is also dealing with a rise in healthcare related costs. Although the Australian government has limited physicians on how much they can be reimbursed for services, there are no regulations preventing physicians from charging patients more. As mentioned, this has unfortunately led many Australians to believe the services that "cost more must be better quality" when, in fact, this is not accurate. Learning from this mistake, the United States government will need to consider taking a more hands-on approach to controlling price set by both those providing care and the companies providing drugs and products. Again, learning from Australia's example, the government should hire medical experts to determine accurate prices for different products and services. Economists can be brought in to determine fluctuation rates based on geographical location and economic contributors, and though it will take time and collaboration, baseline prices can be determined for each product or service. The Centers for Medicare and Medicaid Services already do a similar practice each year when preparing the Schedule of Benefits. However, many practitioners have complained of the authenticity of these prices, mainly because of the cost of acquiring the supplies needed for different procedures. Again, this is why it will be imperative for the government to take more of a "hands-on" approach and ensure that price gouging is not allowed by those providing the healthcare products as well as those providing the services. Transparency will also be key. This connection of products and services with their correlating prices should also come with explanations on how each price is achievable. The more sufficient information provided, the more informed the population will be, and the easier it will be to implement a new policy.

The same, "hands-on" approach will also have to be used with private insurance companies to ensure price gouging and unjust denial of services do not become, or continue to be, a common practice. As previously mentioned, when the PPACA included a required penalty payment for those who did not purchase their own health insurance, this initiative ultimately failed since many people discovered the penalty was a much lower price to pay than the actual cost of healthcare insurance. Another "loophole" people found was purchasing low cost health insurance, so they would not have to pay the penalty. But this, unfortunately, added them to the percent of the population that was underinsured and therefore contributed to more unreimbursed medical services and more healthcare debt. By controlling price gouging and ensuring a quality product (just, quality health coverage), the government can prevent this same type of failed initiative in the future. Again, the government will need to recruit experts in the field of healthcare services, billing, and insurance to determine adequate reimbursement is provided for services and sufficient, but fair, premiums are charged to individuals. Since geographic location affects costs, state and regional experts in the area will also be required. To ensure an easy transition and the support of the majority, this will also require open communication and sufficient justification on restrictions/allowances to be provided to insurance company representatives and general members of the population. One concern for those in the private insurance industry will be the new restructuring of the industry will ultimately lead to less profit for insurance companies, which could lead to company reformation and layoffs. Since there will be new government positions created that will require experts in this area, those who suffer from company layoffs should have the opportunity to apply and have preferential selection to these newly formed government positions. For others, the government will provide its usual unemployment assistance. Again, these extra measures can help ease some of the unrest and tension that comes along with implementing new policies and plans.

Another common problem leading to rising costs in healthcare is unnecessary procedures. This also leads us to addressing the third weakness of the United States' healthcare system that was mentioned: communication gaps. There are numerous accounts of procedures being repeated or unnecessarily ordered due to a lack of communication among providers and/or insurance companies. Unnecessary procedures lead to a waste of materials, time, and resources. Australia suffers from the same weakness with their own lack of coordination of care. In 2009, the United States attempted to address this issue with the introduction of the Health Information Technology for Economic and Clinical Health Act (HITECH Act). The HITECH Act was created to encourage the implementation of health information technology and promote the adoption of electronic health records by healthcare facilities. Although a developed country and known for advanced technology, the United States was more than 10 years behind many other countries in implementing EHRs, jokingly being deemed a "late adapter" by other countries. And though we have seen many positive results from the adaption of EHRs into the healthcare field, the rush and lack of a national implementation plan have led to major problems that have inadvertently added to the lack of communication problem. The EHR industry quickly grew, leading numerous options for companies such as EPIC, Athena, McKesson, Allscripts, Praxis, etc. These systems, unfortunately, do not always communicate, leading to more communication gaps. Since most patients will be treated by different physicians with different specialties, the chances are very high that they will also receive care from different offices and/or facilities. With a plethora of EHR systems to choose from, the chances are even higher that the patient's information will be stored in numerous EHR systems. The inability of the systems to communicate requires patients to provide their information numerous times and increases the chances that vital information will be lost between providers. To address this issue, the government will need to step in and ensure communication between systems. One solution is to require all medical providers to purchase the same system. This solution has many issues, one is the cost. Some systems, such as Epic, have a high cost associated with them but they offer numerous options (i.e., all the "bells and whistles") including the ability to display and store radiological images, lab results, cardiac scans, prescriptions, operating room capabilities, trauma care, etc. This may be great for a hospital, but a small outpatient clinic does not necessarily need all of these services nor can they justify the cost of paying for something they do not necessarily need. Additionally, requiring all healthcare providers to purchase the same EHR would also lead to a monopoly within the industry and cause the loss of jobs for any of those working for the EHR companies who are "not chosen." For a better solution, the government can require all EHR manufacturers to ensure their systems are compatible with interfaces that will allow them to communicate with other EHR systems. An interface is a program that enables different software programs to communicate with one another. By requiring all EHR manufacturers to create systems that are compatible with interfaces that would ensure their communication with other EHR systems, the lack of communication and connection would be resolved. This would also need to be taken a step further to include insurance company systems which, again, would speed up payment processing and reduce the risk of unnecessary or unjustifiable procedures being performed.

CONCLUSION

Much can be learned from one another if we take the time to observe others, praise their successes, and be open to change. No system is perfect, but by combining positive attributes from different systems and learning from the mistakes of others, we can continue to improve and increase the quality of our systems. The United States healthcare system has needed a change for quite some time. However, with a growing population and constant advances in medicine, the healthcare industry has not made sufficient changes to ensure affordable, top quality care for American citizens. Although not perfect, Australia has set a good example with their universal

Medicare system, and has received and continues to receive mostly praise from Australian citizens when asked about their opinions of the universal healthcare system. The United States would benefit from reviewing Australia's Medicare and applying some of the key components.

REFERENCES

Atkinson, J. G., and Giovanis, T. N. (2015). The Patient Protection and Affordable Care Act: Suggestions for Improvements. *American journal of public health, 105*(Suppl 5), S630. doi:10.2105/AJPH.2015.302932

Bhaduri, S. (2020). United States of America: Healthcare System Overview and SWOT Analysis. *The Indian Practitioner, 73*(9), 46–49. http://articles.theindianpractitioner.com/index.php/tip/article/view/1055

Dixit, S. K., & Sambasivan, M. (2018). A review of the Australian healthcare system: A policy perspective. *SAGE Open Medicine, 6*. doi:10.1177/2050312118769211 PMID:29686869

Fix, G. M., VanDeusen Lukas, C., Bolton, R. E., Hill, J. N., Mueller, N., LaVela, S. L., & Bokhour, B. G. (2018). Patient-centred care is a way of doing things: How healthcare employees conceptualize patient-centred care. *Health Expectations, 21*(1), 300–307. doi:10.1111/hex.12615 PMID:28841264

Fryling, M. J., Johnston, C., & Hayes, L. J. (2011). Understanding observational learning: An interbehavioral approach. *Analysis of Verbal Behavior, 27*(1), 191–203. doi:10.1007/BF03393102 PMID:22532764

Robinson, S., Varhol, R., Ramamurthy, V., Denehy, M., Hendrie, D., O'Leary, P., & Selvey, L. (2015). The Australian primary healthcare experiment: A national survey of Medicare Locals. *BMJ Open, 5*(3), e007191. doi:10.1136/bmjopen-2014-007191 PMID:25818276

Straube, B. M. (2013). A Role for Government: An Observation on Federal Healthcare Efforts in Prevention. *American Journal of Preventive Medicine, 44*(1), S39–S42. doi:10.1016/j.amepre.2012.09.009 PMID:23195165

Chapter 11
Public Charge in the Time of Coronavirus

Martha Tepepa
Western Connecticut State University, USA

ABSTRACT

In 2020, the United States government passed legislation and stabilization packages to respond to the COVID-19 outbreak by providing paid sick leave, tax credits, and free virus testing; expanding food assistance and unemployment benefits; and increasing Medicaid funding. However, the response to the global pandemic might have been hindered by the lassitude of the state and the prevailing conception of social policy that leaves the most vulnerable unprotected. The "zero tolerance" immigration campaign that was executed until January 2021 had negative public health consequences, especially for the prevention of communicable diseases. In addition to the systemic obstacles noncitizens face in their access to healthcare, changes to immigration law that penalize recipients of some social services on grounds that they are a public charge further restricted their access to treatment and hindered the fight against the pandemic.

INTRODUCTION

In 2020, the United States government passed legislation and stabilization packages to respond to the COVID-19 (i.e., coronavirus disease 2019) outbreak by providing paid sick leave, tax credits, and free COVID-19 testing; expanding food assistance and unemployment benefits; and increasing Medicaid funding: "Under the Senate Republicans' original bill, individuals could receive one-time checks of a maximum of $1,200 or $2,400 for married couples, plus $500 per child. Those earning more

DOI: 10.4018/978-1-6684-4060-5.ch011

money would get a bigger check and the payment would phase out for those earning more than $75,000, ending entirely for taxpayers with more than $99,000 in income or families earning $198,000," with the initial measure also stating that "it will reduce payments to $600 for people with no income tax liability but at least $2,500 in earnings" (Hulse 2020). Thus, people with lower income levels would receive less cash. Lawmakers from both parties attacked this and, eventually, it was decided that the full amount would be sent to those families as well.

The Coronavirus Aid, Relief, and Economic Security (CARES) Act passed by unanimous vote in the Senate and was signed into law on Friday, March 31, 2020 (the health crisis started in late February, evidence of the lack of direction and unpreparedness of the governing elite). The CARES Act included a delay for the payment of the employer payroll tax –one of the primary funding mechanisms for Social Security– for the rest of 2020. Corporations like airlines, cruise companies, and fossil fuel firms received a $500 billion business relief program "slush fund," controlled by the administration. The population that was already registered with the Internal Revenue Service (IRS) or the Social Security Administration received automatic payments, while those that don't normally file a return with the IRS and/or lack a standard checking account faced more challenges in receiving their check.[1]

The implicit intent of the government's first direct action was to continue ceding all crucial initiatives to the private sector, reinforcing the market's dominance while undercutting the state's strategic intervention, a process evident during the years of the Trump administration, when the reconstruction of Puerto Rico's economy after Hurricane Maria was left to the private sector (Weisbrot 2019). The administration's initial unwillingness to use the Defense Procurement Act to speed up the production of medical equipment necessary to combat the pandemic also demonstrated their aversion to direct market intervention. The retraction of the state's involvement during the pandemic allowed colossal profits for specific industries like biotechnology firms, major pharmaceuticals firms, makers of generic drugs, medical equipment manufacturing firms, and health insurance companies (Assis 2022, Doctors Without Borders 2022, Valinsky 2020).

So far, the question of the virus' impact has been addressed, but one important fact that has not been addressed is the access to treatment for all. Some families might not get their thousand dollars in the mail, but even if they got their check, it would make little difference because most likely they won't have access to treatment if they get sick.

Throughout history, there have been pandemics that wipe out human assumptions of invincibility and reveal the mighty power of tiny pathogens to bring us down without discrimination: poor, rich, white, black, old, young, male, female, and so on.

In *Love in the Time of Cholera*, Nobel Prize-winner Gabriel García Márquez (1988) writes a love story set in a coastal town near the Magdalena River, weaving in details of the epidemic of cholera morbus that ravaged Colombia. The profound inequalities of the region in the nineteenth century, when the story is set, are reflected in the extreme social-spatial division: the great families of European descent (local aristocrats) that occupy the structured downtown and the popular class that inhabits the inner city. The colonial infrastructure is crumbling and Spanish-built sewers discharge waste into the cove, where offal from the slaughterhouse is also thrown away. Nearby, the market operates on top its own garbage heap.

While old colonial mansions have latrines and septic tanks, the black population and outcasts, who represent two-thirds of the population, are relegated to the outskirts where there is no infrastructure. In these communities, not only was breathing lethal, drinking water was also harmful since it was a sanctuary for water worms and lacked the safe chemical composition for human consumption.[2]

In the novel, as in real life, the cholera epidemic does not discriminate in who it infects, but hits the poor much harder than the wealthy, mainly because of their lack of access to sanitary conditions. It is calculated that during the cholera epidemic that blasted Colombian towns along the Caribbean coast in the mid- to late-nineteenth century the mortality rate was 50 percent and over 200,000 people died.

García Márquez said that the novel was his most political and critical of the traditional local power groups. The governing elite seems lethargic, almost immobile, too invested in promoting their noble descent and in their internal fights for power. They are disconnected from the realities of the putrefaction of the city, the overt exploitation of natural resources, and the general deterioration of the environment. The epidemic finds them underprepared and unable to manage a city under siege from a deadly contagion.

EPIDEMICS AND THE STATE

The state is an essential part of the design and implementation of policies that guide the nation's development:

The State assumes a strategic and leading role through a combination of democratic planning within all sectors: the market, the public, the private. [The national development strategy] expresses the will of a hegemonic group and a coalition of forces, with interests, objectives, resources and powers, but capable of coincidences. Through the State, a hegemonic group or coalition, in the conditions and under the determinations of a given society and of a certain phase of its evolution, can mobilize and use a diversity of resources, through its decisions and activities, for the achievement of its conservation or change objectives, in coincidence with a confrontation with other groups of different interests and projects. Development strategies and policies are specified through questions and dilemmas, answers and solutions, establishing balances and combinations (Kaplan 1995: 45-46).

The state provides and satisfies basic needs, mainly related to economic, educational, and health needs, through social policy. The state's actions are the result of the government's conception of social problems and the characteristics of the instruments adopted to tackle them. In some countries, the state is the main guarantor and regulator; in others the action is delegated to the private sector and organizations.

According to Keynes's concept of the Social State, the conjunction of economic growth on the one hand and a better redistribution of wealth on the other –economic development plus social welfare– leads to greater social justice (Wray 2005: 2). Under this approach, one of the main functions of the state is the improvement of the population's general well-being. Thus, extreme poverty in a country is the most acute expression of the fact that the economic and social structure of the state and the ruling government have not satisfied the needs of all (Filgueira 2005: 2).

The conceptualization of the state's action presents different ethical, ideological, and political orientations. Its design mixes a series of actors with different principles and interests, which influence the final result and the type of tools applied: "Ideally, the objective of all social development policies is to put an end to economic inequalities and imbalances, assuming the role of redistributing income in favor of the weakest" (Sen 2003).

The social policy model of the United States can be described as a means-tested assistance model, according to the typology proposed by Esping-Andersen.[3] In this model, the social safety net forces participants to integrate into the market, through policies based on tests of means that offer a minimum coverage with meager benefits. This model strengthens the market's role because everyone is forced to contract private assistance while the state is a mere facilitator that delegates responsibility, production, action, and profits to the private sector. The benefits are scarce and generally associated with social stigma (similar to the Poor Laws in the United Kingdom in the nineteenth century) provoking embarrassment, resentment, or shame. By stigmatizing and punishing participants, the model promotes a dual social system.

For example, families interested in receiving the housing choice voucher program must prove that their family income and assets are below a certain level set by the US Department of Housing and Urban Development (HUD), the program's administrator.[4] The information provided by applicant families is verified by local agencies, employers, and banks. If approved, the amount of housing assistance is calculated based on the rent for a moderately priced dwelling unit in the local market. The family can select a unit with a rent that is below or above the payment standard and "must pay 30 percent of its monthly adjusted gross income for rent and utilities, and if the unit rent is greater than the payment standard the family is required to pay the additional amount" (HUD 2020).

Despite the huge demand for housing assistance, the resources available to HUD and the local housing agencies were cut in the Trump administration's fiscal year 2020 budget request. This action eliminated or deeply cut essential housing and community development programs like the national Housing Trust Fund, the HOME Investments Partnership program, and public housing capital repairs, leaving families in need in waiting lists and facing homelessness: "Overall, the administration proposes to cut HUD by an astounding $9.6 billion or 18 percent below 2019 enacted levels, imposing deep cuts to affordable housing and community development as well as other essential programs that ensure basic living standards" (NLIHC 2020).

Gordon (2004) argues that the orthodox policies in the means-tested assistance model rest on three elements: economic growth, human capital development through education, and a minimum social safety net for the poor. He stresses that the axis on which these types of policies rest –privatization, liberalization of the capital market, and a system of prices controlled by the market and free trade– has, in many countries, led to, among other things, increases in poverty levels. "Countries can open their economies and not generate growth or human development. Russia generated trade and attracted private capital flows with the opening in the 1990s, but economic stagnation and human deprivation are severe. Between 1989 and 1996, men's life expectancy fell by almost four years to 60, two years less than the average for developing countries. The under-five mortality rate is 25 per 1,000 live births, compared to 14 in Poland. In addition, homicides and illegal drug trafficking have increased" (UNDP 1999: 85).

Aside from the limited reach of social policies, the US government's current position on the origin of social problems, as well as on the perception of policy recipients, is to assume that they are product of individual failures –people lacking skills and entrepreneurship– and judging those that fall behind (the poor) as lazy, delinquent, and unworthy of assistance: "the dominant culture [in the United States] spreads the idea that the poor are in that situation because they have certain behaviors resulting from moral deficiencies or a wrong system of values" (Schteingart 1999: 340). Among those not blamed for their situation are women, widows, the disabled, children, and the elderly, often called "vulnerable" population. Ideal citizens are individuals believed to have more potential to make economic contributions and live within their own means without relying on social programs, while those who demonstrate higher employability, consistently demonstrate agency-verified need, or suffer from severe vulnerabilities are considered deserving.

These perceptions, however biased they might be, are the social realities guiding the US government in addressing needs. Ideally, the state's interventions are fact-based and anti-discriminatory. However, under the Trump administration, this was not possible since there were clear prejudices harbored by frontline public sector workers and policy-makers that translated into overt discriminatory treatment of citizens in need, while noncitizens were subjected to a "public charge" consideration.

PUBLIC CHARGE

The word "charge" has many meanings in the Webster's Third New International Dictionary of the English Language, but the one that can be applied unambiguously to a person and best clarifies the phrase "become a public charge" is "a person entrusted to the care, custody, management, or support of the public system." The term has been defined by the United States Department of Justice Immigration and Naturalization Service (INS) as "a complete, or nearly complete, dependence on the Government for subsistence, as demonstrated by either the receipt of public cash assistance for income maintenance or institutionalization for long-term care at Government expense" (INS 1999).

During the early years of the United States, individuals who became dependent on the government were institutionalized in asylums or placed in almshouses for the poor. As the welfare state developed, a model of limited-purpose public assistance was established against the backdrop of the "public charge" concept used in immigration law beginning in the late 1800s.

The term public charge reflects the concept of dependency, rather than solidarity, and has been in use for more than a century. A recent use dates from the 1996 Personal Responsibility and Work Opportunity Reconciliation Act (PRWORA) welfare reform signed by President Clinton, which imposed new restrictions on noncitizens' eligibility for federal, state, and local public benefits. The eligibility restrictions did not include emergency medical assistance; short-term, in-kind, emergency disaster relief; public health assistance related to immunizations and treatment of a communicable disease; certain in-kind services (e.g., soup kitchens, etc.) designated by the attorney general as necessary for the protection of life and safety; and assistance under certain HUD programs.

Though legally eligible, accepting benefits such as cash assistance for income maintenance benefits, including Supplemental Security Income (SSI) and Temporary Assistance for Needy Families (TANF), as well as other state or local cash assistance programs may result in an individual being determined a public charge and affect a noncitizen's right to remain in the United States (a person is also considered a public charge if they are institutionalized at the government's expense, other than imprisonment for conviction of a crime). The rule states that in terms of immigration status, the "aliens" that receive any form of cash assistance for income maintenance or are institutionalized for long-term care are not *necessarily* inadmissible, ineligible to adjust status, or deportable on the grounds that they are a public charge: "… the law requires that a variety of other factors and prerequisites must be considered as well" (INS 1999).

The restrictions led numerous noncitizens to refrain from applying for benefits, fearing the negative consequences of potentially being deemed a public charge.[5] This presents negative public health consequences, especially for the treatment of communicable diseases. If a large segment of the population fears obtaining necessary medical treatment, it will not only cause considerable harm to families but will jeopardize the general public. For example, infectious diseases may spread as a large percentage of the population declines immunization or are refused treatment during a pandemic. This tension between immigration and welfare laws was exacerbated by the changes to immigration laws implemented during the Trump administration.

On February 24, 2020, the Inadmissibility on Public Charge Grounds final rule was implemented nationwide. Citing the basic principle of self-sufficiency in the United States since the earliest immigration waves of the 1800s, the government put into statute that those unable to care for themselves without becoming a public charge were inadmissible in the United States. The final rule required that noncitizens seeking to preserve, extend, or change their immigrant status show that they have not received public benefits (as defined in the rule) over a designated threshold.[6]

CORONAVIRUS

The novel coronavirus first labeled as SARS-CoV2 emerged in Wuhan, China at the end of 2019. The virus quickly spread to all Chinese provinces and the World Health Organization declared the spread of COVID-19 a pandemic on March 11, 2020. As of April 4, 2020, authorities in 206 countries and territories had reported more than 1,134,000 cases. Although countries have taken several actions to contain the virus, the effectiveness of these efforts is unknown due to the uncertainties regarding the pathogen's transmissibility and its virulence. Li et al. (2020) found that a high proportion of undocumented infections, "many of whom were likely not severely symptomatic, appears to have facilitated the rapid spread of the virus throughout China. Indeed, suppression of the infectiousness of these undocumented cases in model simulations reduces the total number of documented cases and the overall spread of SARS-CoV2." Their findings underscore the importance of the state's action and efficiency:

Presently, there are four endemic coronavirus strains currently circulating in human populations (229E, HKU1, NL63, OC43). If the novel coronavirus follows the pattern of 2009 H1N1 pandemic influenza, it will also spread globally and become a fifth endemic coronavirus within the human population... [Our] findings also indicate that a radical increase in the identification and isolation of currently undocumented infections would be needed to fully control SARS-CoV2. Increased news coverage and awareness of the virus in the general population have already likely prompted increased rates of seeking medical care for respiratory symptoms. In addition, awareness among healthcare providers, public health officials and the availability of viral identification assays suggest that capacity for identifying previously missed infections has increased. Further, general population and government response efforts have increased the use of face masks, restricted travel, delayed school reopening and isolated suspected persons, all of which could additionally slow the spread of SARS-CoV2 (Li et al. 2020).

PUBLIC CHARGE AND CORONAVIRUS IN TIMES OF RACISM AND XENOPHOBIA

During disease outbreaks, attacks on marginalized groups are not an exception, but the norm. Racism and xenophobia are enhanced by discourse that targets certain ethnic groups, suggesting they are at fault for spreading the disease or are *free riders* who take resources that should not be available to them. Pandemics increase far-right extremism and prejudiced attitudes toward those who look different. Examples of this are found throughout history, with European colonists blamed for America's smallpox epidemic in the sixteenth century, Jewish communities targeted during the bubonic plague, and Irish immigrants blamed for typhoid in the 1800s.

Immigrants without papers have also been prosecuted for accessing cash assistance, long-term institutionalized care, or medical attention that many believe should be reserved only for citizens. Non-white legal residents are also scrutinized for their use of public services and labeled as undeserving. Refugees are often accused of draining resources and struggle to counter extremist narratives and social distrust in host communities.

Immigration policies in the United States have intensified these sentiments and could undermine efforts to detect and combat the COVID-19. Those apprehended after crossing the border will most likely be put in detention facilities with poor conditions, such as crowded and cramped environments, that are detrimental to epidemic management. Immigrants without papers, already in the United States, might not seek care out of fear of deportation. Parents that might be infected will likely prefer to avoid scrutiny and keep working, thereby increasing the chance of spreading the virus.

The previous administration's "zero tolerance" immigration campaign was an obstacle to treatment and hindered the fight against the pandemic. In the time of COVID-19, these additional attacks leave migrants at a disadvantage when facing segregationist measures such as "English only" policies meant to expel languages other than English from the public sphere. For example, in Arizona, where 30 percent of the residents are Hispanic, the state's department of health services had a portal with updated information about the pandemic, but there was nothing in Spanish. This translates into lack of information for non-English speakers, as a large number of people who do not read in English did not receive information and directions to take precautions to reduce the danger of being infected. Furthermore, families won't be prepared in case they get sick or if the government orders confinement. Nuzzo (2018) studied a mumps outbreak in an immigrant community in Pennsylvania where many people in the community spoke little or no English, and some did not have health insurance or official immigration documentation. The study found that the outbreak was exacerbated because some cases and their contacts may have been deterred from seeking care since they were afraid to be identified as "undocumented immigrants" and be reported to immigration officials.

PUBLIC CHARGE, SOCIAL POLICY, AND COVID-19

At the peak of the pandemic, the of the United States Citizenship and Immigration Services (USCIS 2020) encouraged "all those, including aliens, with symptoms that resemble Coronavirus Disease 2019 (COVID-19) (fever, cough, shortness of breath) seek necessary medical treatment or preventive services. Such treatment or preventive services will not negatively affect any alien as part of a future Public Charge analysis."

The website also stressed that the Public Charge Grounds final rule, implemented on February 24, 2020,[7] "does not restrict noncitizens' access to testing, screening, or treatment of COVID-19 through public sources and to a vaccine, if ever devised, to combat the virus –critical to defending and protecting Americans' health and its healthcare resources."

The text of the Public Charge rule signals that the receipt of public benefits through public treatment or paid by Medicaid, for example, might be considered when weighing the immigration status of noncitizens, thus encouraging noncitizens to use the resources offered by the private sector and discouraging them to apply for or accept public aid even if they desperately need it. The rule also mentioned the consequences of social distancing or quarantine to prevent the spread of COVID-19.

Since noncitizens might be prevented from working or attending school, some might have relied on public benefits for the duration of the outbreak and recovery phase. Thus, under the rule, noncitizens had to provide an explanation and relevant supporting documentation. USCIS then would determine if the submission was relevant and credible, and if it would be considered in the process of adjudicating any application or petition for extension of nonimmigrant stay or change of nonimmigrant status.

Labeling those that receive social programs and benefits as public charge not only labels people but "deservedness" shapes service and policy responses toward them. The term public charge involves perceptions that are distinct from the formal assertion of rights or policies, and informs the decisions that are made about access to public services. During the time of the COVID-19 pandemic, even when noncitizens are granted legal or policy rights to healthcare, these could be denied by frontline health staff if they are not perceived as deserving of care. The health implications for mobile populations subjected to this kind of discrimination can be profound, and during any epidemic can have a serious impact beyond "defending and protecting Americans' health" (USCIS 2020).

CONCLUSION

The actions of the United States government through the pandemic will be less than optimally effective if they don't reach typically overlooked groups, and if they don't acknowledge that public panic and fear –fueled by xenophobia and racist discourse– can be detrimental during a public health emergency. When the state renounces the role of providing basic services for the well-being of its citizens, it leaves the door open for the private sector and other entities to profit from the supply of strategic services during crucial times.

Migration is a human phenomenon that brings a discussion of key human values: dignity, compassion, and respect. An elitist, racist, and cruel society is a nation drained of human values where corporations deserve more than humans. When a country, instead, shows concern for everyone, in taking care of them, it grows. During a similar emergency, the Great Depression, through President Roosevelt's guidance, the state restored public confidence by guaranteeing that the people most affected were able to get back on their feet. While the private sector had a role, the state corrected the imbalance created by ruthless capitalism (Moley 1966). COVID-19 has exposed the difference between social solidarity in the face of the epidemic and social violence in the absence of a public health system that has been privatized to enrich those with a financial advantage, due to political corruption.

REFERENCES

Assis, C. (2022). Amgen stocks rises after COVID drugs boost Q4 profit. *Market Watch.* https://www.marketwatch.com/story/amgen-stock-rises-after-covid-drugs-boost-q4-profit-2022-02-07

Doctors without Borders. (2022). *Moderna posts billions in profit from COVID-19 vaccine but won't share technology*. Doctors Without Boarders https://www.doctorswithoutborders.org/what-we-do/news-stories/news/moderna-posts-billions-profit-covid-19-vaccine-wont-share-technology.

Filgueira, F., Molina, C. G., Papadópulos, J., & Tobar, F. (2005). Universalismo básico: una alternativa posible y necesaria para mejorar las condiciones de vida en América Latina. In C. Molina (Ed.), *Universalismo básico: Una nueva política social para América Latina*. Banco Interamericano de Desarrollo, Editorial Planeta.

Gordon, D. (2004). The International measurement of poverty and anti-poverty policies. In P. Townsend & D. Gordon (Eds.), *World Poverty: New Policies to Defeat an Old Enemy* (2nd ed.). The Policy Press.

Graetz, M., & Shapiro, I. (2020). *The Wolf at the Door: The Menace of Economic Insecurity and How to Fight It*. Harvard University Press.

HUD (US Department of Housing and Urban Development). (2020). Housing Choice Vouchers Fact Sheet. [Data set]. https://www.hud.gov/topics/housing_choice_voucher_program_section_8 .

INS (United States Department of Justice Immigration and Naturalization Service). (1999). Proposed Rule on Inadmissibility and Deportability on Public Charge Grounds; Field Guidance on Deportability and Inadmissibility on Public Charge Grounds; Proposed Rule and Notice. *Federal Register*, *64*(101).

Kandel, W. (2021). The Trump Administration's "Zero Tolerance" Immigration Enforcement Policy. *Congressional Research Service R45266*. https://sgp.fas.org/crs/homesec/R45266.pdf

Kaplan, M. (1995). Teoría y realidad del Estado en América Latina. In M. Mols and J. Thesings (eds.), El Estado en América Latina. Fundación Konrad Adenauer.

Lee, M. (2020). Coronavirus fears show how 'model minority' Asian Americans become the 'yellow peril. *NBC News, Self-Explanatory blog*. https://www.nbcnews.com/think/opinion/coronavirus-fears-show-how-model-minority-asian-americans-become-yellow-ncna1151671 .

Li, R., Sen Pei, B. C., Song, Y., Zhang, T., Yang, W., & Shaman, J. (2020). Substantial undocumented infection facilitates the rapid dissemination of novel coronavirus (SARS-CoV2). *Science Magazine.* http://science.sciencemag.org/content/early/2020/03/13/science.abb3221.abstract

Márquez, G. G. (1988). Love in the Time of Cholera. 1st American ed., Edith Grossman, trans. New York: Alfred A. Knopf.

McFadyen, J. (2020) Immigrants and Public Benefits. *ThoughtCo.* https://www.thoughtco.com/immigrants-and-public-benefits-1951828.

Moley, R. (1966). *The First New Deal.* Harcourt, Brace & World, Inc.

NLIHC (National Low Income Housing Coalition). (2020). President Trump Proposes Drastic Cuts to Affordable Housing Programs. *Analysis of President Trump's FY2020 Budget Request.* https://nlihc.org/resource/analysis-president-trumps-fy2020-budget-request

Nuzzo, J. (2019). Responding to a Mumps Outbreak in a Hard-to-Reach Community. In *Outbreak Observatory Report.* John's Hopkins Bloomberg School of Public Health. https://www.outbreakobservatory.org/outbreakthursday-1/10/10/2019/responding-to-a-mumps-outbreak-in-a-hard-to-reach-community.

Schteingart, M. (1999). *Políticas Sociales para los Pobres en América Latina.* Miguel Ángel Porrúa.

Sen, Amartya. (2003). La economía política de la focalización. *Comercio Exterior, 53*(6).

Simons, M. (1988). García Márquez on Love, Plagues and Politics. *The New York Times.*

UN (United Nations). (2003). The Challenge of Slums. In *United Nations Human Settlements Program 2003 Global Report on Human Settlements. London and Sterling*. Earthscan Publications.

UNDP. (United Nations Development Program) (1999). Human Development Report. Oxford University Press.

USCIS (United States Citizenship and Immigration Services). (2020). Public Charge Fact Sheet. https://www.uscis.gov/news/fact-sheets/public-charge-fact-sheet .

Valinsky, J. (2020). Estas 14 compañías han crecido durante la pandemia de coronavirus. *CNN Espanol.* https://cnnespanol.cnn.com/2020/05/07/estas-14-companias-han-crecido-durante-la-pandemia-de-coronavirus/

Weisbrot, M. (2019). Puerto Rico's Botched Disaster Relief, Unsustainable Debt, and Economic Failure Linked to its Colonial Status. In *CEPR article, May 30*. Center for Economic and Policy Research. https://www.cepr.net/puerto-rico-s-botched-disaster-relief-unsustainable-debt-and-economic-failure-linked-to-its-colonial-status/

Wray, L. R. (2005). Social Security's 70th Anniversary: Surviving 20 Years of Reform. In *Policy Note 2005/6. Annandale-on-Hudson*. Levy Economics Institute of Bard College.

ENDNOTES

1 Graetz and Shapiro (2020) have shown that families receiving government aid are usually unbanked. Their use of debit cards, check-cashing facilities, and payday loan operations is common since they don't maintain a bank account. An additional hurdle is that many states make qualifying for and receiving benefits difficult.

2 This description is sadly valid today for many irregular settlements through Latin America and Asia. As of 2020, many communities have inadequate access to safe and potable water; inadequate access to healthcare infrastructure; precarious and low-quality housing; high levels of overcrowding; and undetermined legal property and residential status (UN 2003).

3 Also called residual or liberal.

4 The housing choice voucher program "is the federal government's major program for assisting very low-income families, the elderly, and the disabled to afford decent, safe, and sanitary housing in the private market. Since housing assistance is provided on behalf of the family or individual, participants are able to find their own housing, including single-family homes, townhouses and apartments" HUD (2020).

5 Although the Public Charge rule assures that noncitizens won't be automatically deemed public charge, it leaves open the possibility that receiving aid might impact their status later: "The rule will provide rules of decision that will apply in proceedings before the Executive Office for Immigration Review (EOIR), as well as proceedings before the Service. The Department anticipates, based on the Service's consultations, that the State Department will adopt the same view and will issue guidance to consular officers accordingly" (INS 1999).

6 The Public Charge Final Rule stopped applying to all pending applications and petitions on March 9, 2021: "On March 9, 2021, the U.S. Court of Appeals for the Seventh Circuit lifted its stay of the U.S. District Court for the Northern District of Illinois' Nov. 2, 2020, decision vacating the Public Charge Final

Rule nationwide." This means that applicants and petitioners no longer have to provide information related to the Public Charge Final Rule. The content related to the 2019 Public Charge Final Rule that affected USCIS forms was removed and USCIS has published new form editions for affected forms.

7 On their website, USCIS states "the Inadmissibility on Public Charge Grounds final rule will be implemented in the United States on Feb. 24, 2020, except in Illinois, where the rule remains enjoined by a federal court as of Jan. 30, 2020. The final rule will apply only to applications and petitions postmarked (or submitted electronically) on or after Feb. 24, 2020" (USCIS 2020).

Compilation of References

S.109 - Pharmacy and Medically Underserved Areas Enhancement Act, 115th Congress (2017-2018). Available at: www.congress.gov/bill/115th-congress/senate-bill/109

H.R. 2759 - Pharmacy and Medically Underserved Areas Enhancement Act, 117th Congress (2021-2022). Available at: www.congress.gov/bill/117th-congress/house-bill/2759

S.1362 - Pharmacy and Medically Underserved Areas Enhancement Act, 117th Congress (2021-2022). Available at: www.congress.gov/bill/117th-congress/senate-bill/1362

Health Resources and Services Administration, U.S. Department of Health and Human Services. (n.d.). *What is Shortage Designation?* Available at: bhw.hrsa.gov/workforce-shortage-areas/shortage-designation

H.R. 7213 - Equitable Community Access to Pharmacist Services Act, 117th Congress (2021-2022). Available at: www.congress.gov/bill/117th-congress/house-bill/7213

U.S. Centers for Disease Control and Prevention. (n.d.a). *The federal retail pharmacy program for COVID-19 vaccination.* Available at: www.cdc.gov/vaccines/covid-19/retail-pharmacy-program/index.html

Harper, P. C. (2015). Pharmacist provider status legislation: Projections and prospects. *Journal of the American Pharmaceutical Association*, *55*(2), 203–207. doi:10.1331/JAPhA.2015.14176 PMID:25749265

Public Law 108-173, Medicare Prescription Drug, Improvement, and Modernization Act of 2003, 108th Congress (2003-2004). Available at: www.govinfo.gov/app/details/PLAW-108publ173

Bluml, B. M. (2005). Definition of medication therapy management: Development of professionwide consensus. *Journal of the American Pharmaceutical Association*, *45*(5), 566–572. doi:10.1331/1544345055001274 PMID:16295641

Viswanathan, M., Kahwati, L. C., Golin, C. E., Blalock, S., Coker-Schwimmer, E., Posey, R., & Lohr, K. N. (2014). *Medication Therapy Management Interventions in Outpatient Settings. Agency for Healthcare Research and Quality (US).* Available at: www.ncbi.nlm.nih.gov/books/NBK294478

The World Bank. (2022). *Databank: World Development Indicators*. https://databank.worldbank.org/reports.aspx?source=World-Development-Indicators

U.S. Social Security Administration. Compilation of the Social Security Laws, Sec. 1861. [42 U.S.C. 1395x]. Available at: www.ssa.gov/OP_Home/ssact/title18/1861.htm

Viswanathan, M., Kahwati, L. C., Golin, C. E., Blalock, S. J., Coker-Schwimmer, E., Posey, R., & Lohr, K. N. (2015). Medication therapy management interventions in outpatient settings: A systematic review and meta-analysis. *JAMA Internal Medicine*, *175*(1), 76–87. doi:10.1001/jamainternmed.2014.5841 PMID:25401788

Pinto, S. L., Kumar, J., Partha, G., & Bechtol, R. A. (2013). Improving the economic and humanistic outcomes for diabetic patients: Making a case for employer-sponsored medication therapy management. *ClinicoEconomics and Outcomes Research*, *5*, 153–159. PMID:23610526

Pellegrin, K. L., Krenk, L., Oakes, S. J., Ciarleglio, A., Lynn, J., McInnis, T., Bairos, A. W., Gomez, L., McCrary, M. B., Hanlon, A. L., & Miyamura, J. (2017). Reductions in medication-related hospitalizations in older adults with medication management by hospital and community pharmacists: A quasi-experimental study. *Journal of the American Geriatrics Society*, *65*(1), 212–219. doi:10.1111/jgs.14518 PMID:27714762

Tichy, E. M., Hoffman, J. M., Suda, K. J., Rim, M. H., Tadrous, M., Cuellar, S., Clark, J. S., Ward, J., & Schumock, G. T. (2022). National trends in prescription drug expenditures and projections for 2022. *American Journal of Health-System Pharmacy*, *79*(14), 1158–1172. doi:10.1093/ajhp/zxac102 PMID:35385103

Academy of Managed Care Pharmacy. (n.d.). *Specialty Pharmaceuticals, Concepts in Managed Care Pharmacy, Managed Care Pharmacy 101*. Available at: www.amcp.org/about/managed-care-pharmacy-101/concepts-managed-care-pharmacy/specialty-pharmaceuticals

Advisory Committee on Immunization Practices (ACIP), U.S. Centers for Disease Control and Prevention. (n.d.). *ACIP Vaccine Recommendations and Guidelines*. Available at: https://www.cdc.gov/vaccines/hcp/acip-recs/index.html

U.S. Centers for Disease Control and Prevention. (n.d.b). *Immunization Schedules*. Available at: www.cdc.gov/vaccines/schedules

U.S. Food and Drug Administration. (n.d.a). *Vaccines licensed for use in the United States*. Available at: www.fda.gov/vaccines-blood-biologics/vaccines/vaccines-licensed-use-united-states

Dooling, K. L., Guo, A., Patel, M., Lee, G. M., Moore, K., Belongia, E. A., & Harpaz, R. (2018). Recommendations of the Advisory Committee on Immunization Practices for use of herpes zoster vaccines. *MMWR. Morbidity and Mortality Weekly Report*, *67*(3), 103–108. doi:10.15585/mmwr.mm6703a5 PMID:29370152

Terlizzi, E. P., & Black, L. I. (2020). *Shingles vaccination among adults aged 60 and over: United States, 2018. NCHS Data Brief, no 370*. National Center for Health Statistics.

Braithwaite, J. (2018). Changing how we think about healthcare improvement. *BMJ (Clinical Research Ed.), 361*, k2014. doi:10.1136/bmj.k2014 PMID:29773537

Bureau of Labor Statistics, U.S. Department of Labor. (n.d.). *Occupational Outlook Handbook, Pharmacists.* Available at: www.bls.gov/ooh/healthcare/pharmacists.htm

Bacci, J. L., Hansen, R., Ree, C., Reynolds, M. J., Stergachis, A., & Odegard, P. S. (2019). The effects of vaccination forecasts and value-based payment on adult immunizations by community pharmacists. *Vaccine, 37*(1), 152–159. doi:10.1016/j.vaccine.2018.11.018 PMID:30446177

American Pharmacists Association and National Alliance of State Pharmacy Associations. (2022). *Pharmacist administered vaccines.* Available at: www.pharmacist.com/DNNGlobalStorageRedirector.ashx?egsfid=EACvwV2aS-8%3d

American Pharmacists Association. (n.d.b). *Guidelines for Pharmacy-based Immunization Advocacy and Administration.* Available at: aphanet.pharmacist.com/sites/default/files/files/Guidelines_for_Pharmacy_Based_IMZ_Advocacy_Approved_Jan_26_2019.pdf

Isenor, J. E., Edwards, N. T., Alia, T. A., Slayter, K. L., MacDougall, D. M., McNeil, S. A., & Bowles, S. K. (2016). Impact of pharmacists as immunizers on vaccination rates: A systematic review and meta-analysis. *Vaccine, 34*(47), 5708–5723. doi:10.1016/j.vaccine.2016.08.085 PMID:27765379

Baroy, J., Chung, D., Frisch, R., Apgar, D., & Slack, M. K. (2016). The impact of pharmacist immunization programs on adult immunization rates: A systematic review and meta-analysis. *Journal of the American Pharmaceutical Association, 56*(4), 418–426. doi:10.1016/j.japh.2016.03.006 PMID:27450138

U.S. Centers for Medicare and Medicaid Services. (n.d.). *Part D Enhanced Medication Therapy Management Model.* Available at: innovation.cms.gov/innovation-models/enhancedmtm

U.S. Administration for Strategic Preparedness and Response. (n.d.). *Test to Treat.* Available at: aspr.hhs.gov/TestToTreat/Pages/default.aspx

U.S. Food and Drug Administration. (n.d.b). *Coronavirus (COVID-19) update: FDA authorizes pharmacists to prescribe Paxlovid with certain limitations.* Available at: www.fda.gov/news-events/press-announcements/coronavirus-covid-19-update-fda-authorizes-pharmacists-prescribe-paxlovid-certain-limitations

Frost, T. P., & Adams, A. J. (2018). Are advanced practice pharmacist designations really advanced? *Research in Social & Administrative Pharmacy, 14*(5), 501–504. doi:10.1016/j.sapharm.2017.10.002 PMID:29097045

California State Board of Pharmacy. (n.d.). *Advanced Practice Pharmacist information.* Available at: www.pharmacy.ca.gov/applicants/app.shtml

Berenbrok, L. A., Tang, S., Gabriel, N., Guo, J., Sharareh, N., Patel, N., Dickson, S., & Hernandez, I. (2022). Access to community pharmacies: A nationwide geographic information systems cross-sectional analysis. *Journal of the American Pharmacists Association, 62*(6), 1816–1822.e2. Advance online publication. doi:10.1016/j.japh.2022.07.003 PMID:35965233

Heathcare Tech Outlook. (2020), How Technology is Helping HeathCare System to Improve Care. *Healthcare Tech.* https://www.healthcaretechoutlook.com/news/how-technology-is-helping-healthcare-system-to-improve-care-nid-1942.html

American Medical Association. (2020). *AMA opposes expanding pharmacists' ability to provide child vaccines.* Press release. Available at: www.ama-assn.org/press-center/press-releases/ama-opposes-expanding-pharmacists-ability-provide-child-vaccines

American Medical Association. (2022a). *AMA statement on Administration's test-to-treat COVID-19 plan.* Press release. Available at: www.ama-assn.org/press-center/press-releases/ama-statement-administration-s-test-treat-covid-19-plan

Madara, J. (2022). *Letter to Representatives Kind and McKinley.* Available at: searchltf.ama-assn.org/letter/documentDownload?uri=%2Funstructured%2Fbinary%2Fletter%2FLETTERS%2F2022-4-12-Letter-to-Kind-and-McKinley-re-HR-7213-Equitable-Community-Access-to-Pharmacists-v3.pdf

American Medical Association. (2022b). AMA statement on Paxlovid prescribing. Press release. Available at: www.ama-assn.org/press-center/press-releases/ama-statement-paxlovid-prescribing

American Pharmacists Association. (2022a). *APhA House of Delegates passes policy addressing access to pharmacist-provided services.* Available at: www.pharmacist.com/Pharmacy-News/apha-house-of-delegates-passes-policy-addressing-access-to-pharmacist-provided-services

American Pharmacists Association. (2022b). *APhA addresses AMA's inaccurate description of H.R. 7213 and viewpoints of most physicians working alongside pharmacists.* Press release. Available at: www.pharmacist.com/APhA-Press-Releases/apha-addresses-amas-inaccurate-description-of-hr-7213-and-viewpoints-of-most-physicians-working-alongside-pharmacists

Blank, C. (2022). *Pharmacy groups respond to AMA criticism on pharmacists prescribing Paxlovid.* Available at: www.drugtopics.com/view/pharmacy-groups-respond-to-ama-criticism-on-pharmacists-prescribing-paxlovid

Walgreen Co. (2022). *Walgreens now providing Pfizer and Moderna COVID-19 vaccines to children ages 3 and older at select locations nationwide.* Available at: news.walgreens.com/press-center/news/walgreens-now-providing-pfizer-and-moderna-covid-19-vaccines-to-children-ages-3-and-older-at-select-locations-nationwide.htm

Liu, Y. (2022). Passion and purpose drive the 2022 APhA House of Delegates sessions. APhA–APRS, The potential impact on science and research. *Journal of the American Pharmaceutical Association, 62*(4), 918–919. doi:10.1016/j.japh.2022.05.023

American Pharmacists Association. (n.d.a). *Pharmacy's Top Priority: Medicare Provider Status Recognition.* Available at: www.pharmacist.com/Advocacy/Issues/Medicare-Provider-Status-Recognition

Gilbert, A. W., Billany, J. C., Adam, R., Martin, L., Tobin, R., Bagdai, S., Galvin, N., Farr, I., Allain, A., Davies, L., & Bateson, J. (2020). Rapid implementation of virtual clinics due to COVID-19: Report and early evaluation of a quality improvement initiative. *BMJ Open Quality*, *9*(2), e000985. doi:10.1136/bmjoq-2020-000985 PMID:32439740

American Society of Health-System Pharmacists. (n.d.). *Provider Status Readiness*. Available at: www.ashp.org/pharmacy-practice/resource-centers/provider-status-readiness

Future of Pharmacy Care Coalition. (n.d.). Available at: pharmacycare.org/support/

H.R. 592 - Pharmacy and Medically Underserved Areas Enhancement Act, 114th Congress (2015-2016). Available at: www.congress.gov/bill/114th-congress/house-bill/592

S.314 - Pharmacy and Medically Underserved Areas Enhancement Act, 114th Congress (2015-2016). Available at: www.congress.gov/bill/114th-congress/senate-bill/314

H.R. 592 - Pharmacy and Medically Underserved Areas Enhancement Act, 115th Congress (2017-2018). Available at: www.congress.gov/bill/115th-congress/house-bill/592

Ackerman, B. G. (2019, April 17). Is the Doctor In? Medical Malpractice Issues in the Age of Telemedicine. *The National Law Review*. https://www.natlawreview.com/article/doctor-medical-malpractice-issues-age-telemedicine

Aetna. (2021). *Get started with telemedicine*. Aetna. https://www.aetna.com/individuals-families/member-rights-resources/covid19/telemedicine.html

Agency for Healthcare Research and Quality. (2020, October). *CAHPS Health Plan Survey.* AHRQ. https://www.ahrq.gov/cahps/surveys-guidance/hp/index.html

Agency for Healthcare Research and Quality. (2020, September). *How to Obtain Consent for Telehealth.* AHRQ. https://www.ahrq.gov/health-literacy/improve/informed-consent/obtain.html

AHA. (2011). *Heart Disease and Stroke Statistics* [Data set]. American Heart Association.

Andriola, M. (2019). Telemedicine and Legal Disruption. *Health Law & Policy Brief*, *13*(2), [iii]-30. https://heinonline.org/HOL/P?h=hein.journals/heallaw13&i=73

Aronson, S. H. (1977). The Lancet on the Telephone 1876-1975. *Medical History*, *21*(1), 69–87. doi:10.1017/S0025727300037182 PMID:320411

Arrow, K. (1963). Uncertainty and the Welfare Economics of Medical Care. *The American Economic Review*, *3*(5), 941–973. https://www.jstor.org/stable/1812044

Assis, C. (2022). Amgen stocks rises after COVID drugs boost Q4 profit. *Market Watch.* https://www.marketwatch.com/story/amgen-stock-rises-after-covid-drugs-boost-q4-profit-2022-02-07

Atkinson, J. G., and Giovanis, T. N. (2015). The Patient Protection and Affordable Care Act: Suggestions for Improvements. *American journal of public health, 105*(Suppl 5), S630. doi:10.2105/AJPH.2015.302932

Badaracco, A. (n.d.). *Medicaid State Plan Fee-for-Service Payments for Services Delivered Via Telehealth.* Medicaid. https://www.medicaid.gov/medicaid/benefits/downloads/medicaid-telehealth-services.pdf

Barr, N. (1992, June). Economic Theory and the Welfare State: A Survey and Interpretation. *Journal of Economic Literature, 30*(2), 741–803.

Bashshur, R. e., Doarn, C. R., Frenk, J. M., Kvedar, J. C., & Woolliscroft, J. O. (2020). Telemedicine and the COVID-19 Pandemic, Lessons for the Future. *Telemedicine Journal and e-Health, 26*(5), 571–573. doi:10.1089/tmj.2020.29040.rb PMID:32275485

Baumann, P. K., & Scales, T. (2016). *History of Information Communication Technology and Telehealth.* Winston-Salem State University. https://search-proquest-com.courseinfo.wssu.edu/docview/1863562170?pq-origsite=summon

Berg, J. (2014). The E-Health Revolution and the Necessary Evolution of Informed Consent. *Indiana Health Law Review.* https://heinonline.org/HOL/P?h=hein.journals/inhealr11&i=597

Bhaduri, S. (2020). United States of America: Healthcare System Overview and SWOT Analysis. *The Indian Practitioner, 73*(9), 46–49. http://articles.theindianpractitioner.com/index.php/tip/article/view/1055

Board on Health Care Services. (2012, November 20). *The Role of Telehealth in an Evolving Health Care Environment: Workshop Summary.* Institute of Medicine. https://www.ncbi.nlm.nih.gov/books/NBK207141/#_NBK207141_pubdet_

Bortniker, F., & Warren, A. (2020, April 15). *COVID-19: Resources for Oncology Providers (Telehealth, Clinical Trials, Reporting Deadlines).* Winston-Salem State University. https://search-proquest-com.courseinfo.wssu.edu/docview/2389842056/126488F7309143FEPQ/3?accountid=15070

Center for Connected Health Policy. (2020). *State Telehealth Laws & Reimbursement Policies.* CCHPCA. https://www.cchpca.org/sites/default/files/2020-10/CCHP%2050%20STATE%20REPORT%20FALL%202020%20FINAL.pdf

Centers for Disease Control and Prevention. (2018, September 14). *Health Insurance Portability and Accountability Act of 1996 (HIPAA).* CDC. https://www.cdc.gov/phlp/publications/topic/hipaa.html

Centers for Disease Control and Prevention. (2019). *Health Insurance Portability and Accountability Act of 1996 (HIPAA).* CDC. https://www.cdc.gov/phlp/publications/topic/hipaa.html

Centers for Medicare and Medicaid Services. (2020). *Rural Health Council.* CMS. https://www.cms.gov/About-CMS/Agency-Information/OMH/equity-initiatives/rural-health/rural-health-council

Centers for Medicare and Medicaid Services. (2020, February 19). *COVID-19 Emergency Declaration Blanket Waivers for Health Care Providers.* CMS. https://www.cms.gov/files/document/covid-19-emergency-declaration-waivers.pdf

Centers for Medicare and Medicaid Services. (2020, March 17). *Medicare Telemedicine Health Care Provider Fact Sheet.* CMS. https://www.cms.gov/newsroom/fact-sheets/medicare-telemedicine-health-care-provider-fact-sheet

Centers for Medicare and Medicaid Services. (n.d.). *List of Telehealth Services.* CMS. https://www.cms.gov/Medicare/Medicare-General-Information/Telehealth/Telehealth-Codes

Christensen, C. (2012). *Disruptive Innovation.* Clayton Christensen. https://claytonchristensen.com/key-concepts/

Christensen, C. M. (2011). *Disrupting College.* Center for American Progress: https://www.americanprogress.org/issues/economy/reports/2011/02/08/9034/disrupting-college/

Christensen, C. M. (2015, December 1). What Is Disruptive Innovation? *Harvard Business Review.* https://hbr.org/2015/12/what-is-disruptive-innovation

CMS.gov. (2020, December 1). *Trump Administration Finalizes Permanent Expansion of Medicare Telehealth Services and Improved Payment for Time Doctors Spend with Patients.* CMS. https://www.cms.gov/newsroom/press-releases/trump-administration-finalizes-permanent-expansion-medicare-telehealth-services-and-improved-payment

CMS.gov. (2020, October 28). *Rural Health Council.* CMS. https://www.cms.gov/About-CMS/Agency-Information/OMH/equity-initiatives/rural-health/rural-health-council

Department of Health and Human Services Office of Inspector General. (2018, April). *CMS Paid Practitioners for Telehealth Services That Did Not Meet Medicare Requirements.* Garner Health News. http://garnerhealth.com/wp-content/uploads/2014/02/51600058.pdf

DHHS Office of Inspector General. (2020, March 17). *OIG Policy Statement Regarding Physicians and Other Practitioners That Reduce or Waive Amounts Owed by Federal Health Care Program Beneficiaries for Telehealth Services During the 2019 Novel Coronavirus (COVID-19) Outbreak.* OIG. https://oig.hhs.gov/fraud/docs/alertsandbulletins/2020/policy-telehealth-2020.pdf

Dinesen, B. e., Nonnecke, B., Lindeman, D., Toft, E., Kidholm, K., Jethwani, K., Young, H. M., Spindler, H., Oestergaard, C. U., Southard, J. A., Gutierrez, M., Anderson, N., Albert, N. M., Han, J. J., & Nesbitt, T. (2016). Personalized Telehealth in the Future: A Global Research Agenda. *Journal of Medical Internet Research, 18*(3), e53. doi:10.2196/jmir.5257 PMID:26932229

Dixit, S. K., & Sambasivan, M. (2018). A review of the Australian healthcare system: A policy perspective. *SAGE Open Medicine, 6*. doi:10.1177/2050312118769211 PMID:29686869

Doctors without Borders. (2022). *Moderna posts billions in profit from COVID-19 vaccine but won't share technology*. Doctors Without Boarders https://www.doctorswithoutborders.org/what-we-do/news-stories/news/moderna-posts-billions-profit-covid-19-vaccine-wont-share-technology.

eVisit. (2021). *History of Telemedicine*. eVisit. https://evisit.com/resources/history-of-telemedicine/

Fair Health, Inc. (2020). *States by the Numbers*. Fair Health. https://www.fairhealth.org/states-by-the-numbers/telehealth

Federal Office of Rural Health Policy. (2017). *Official web site of the U.S. Health Resources & Services Administration*. Health Resources and Services Administration. https://www.hrsa.gov/rural-health/index.html

Federation of State Medical Boards. (2018). *Covid-19*. FSMB. https://www.fsmb.org/advocacy/covid-19/

Filgueira, F., Molina, C. G., Papadópulos, J., & Tobar, F. (2005). Universalismo básico: una alternativa posible y necesaria para mejorar las condiciones de vida en América Latina. In C. Molina (Ed.), *Universalismo básico: Una nueva política social para América Latina*. Banco Interamericano de Desarrollo, Editorial Planeta.

Fisher, M. (2020, March 19). *Covid-19's Impact on Telehealth & HIPAA Regulations*. Winston-Salem State University. https://search-proquest-com.courseinfo.wssu.edu/docview/2379060880?pq-origsite=summon

Fix, G. M., VanDeusen Lukas, C., Bolton, R. E., Hill, J. N., Mueller, N., LaVela, S. L., & Bokhour, B. G. (2018). Patient-centred care is a way of doing things: How healthcare employees conceptualize patient-centred care. *Health Expectations*, *21*(1), 300–307. doi:10.1111/hex.12615 PMID:28841264

Foley & Lardner. LLP. (2017). *2017 Telemedicine and Digital Health Survey*. Foley. https://www.foley.com/en/files/uploads/2017-Telemedicine-Survey-Report-11-8-17.pdf

Foley & Lardner. LLP. (2021). *Telehealth21 Summit Virtual Conference*. Foley. https://www.foley.com/en/insights/events/2021/03/telehealth21-summit-virtual-conference

Fryling, M. J., Johnston, C., & Hayes, L. J. (2011). Understanding observational learning: An interbehavioral approach. *Analysis of Verbal Behavior*, *27*(1), 191–203. doi:10.1007/BF03393102 PMID:22532764

Gordon, D. (2004). The International measurement of poverty and anti-poverty policies. In P. Townsend & D. Gordon (Eds.), *World Poverty: New Policies to Defeat an Old Enemy* (2nd ed.). The Policy Press.

Graetz, M., & Shapiro, I. (2020). *The Wolf at the Door: The Menace of Economic Insecurity and How to Fight It*. Harvard University Press.

Hadjimatheou, G. (1994). In P. Arestis & M. Sawyer (Eds.), *"Public Expenditure," in The Elgar Companion to Radical Political Economy* (pp. 319–323). Edward Elgar.

Harwell, G. A., Karagiannis, N., & Madjd-Sadjadi, Z. (2013). A Production-oriented Strategy for the United States: A Framework of Alternative Developmentalist Notions. In N. Karagiannis, Z. Madjd-Sadjadi, & S. Sen (Eds.), *The US Economy and Neoliberalism: Alternative Strategies and Policies* (pp. 115–143). Routledge.

Health IT gov. (2019, April 15). *Are there state licensing issues related to telehealth?* The Office of the National Coordinator for Health Information Teaching. https://www.healthit.gov/faq/are-there-state-licensing-issues-related-telehealth

Health Resources & Services Administration. (2021, January). *Telehealth Programs.* HRSA. https://www.hrsa.gov/rural-health/telehealth

Health, F. A. I. R. (2021, March 2). The Impact of COVID-19 on Pediatric Mental Health. *Fair Health.* https://s3.amazonaws.com/media2.fairhealth.org/whitepaper/asset/The%20Impact%20of%20COVID-19%20on%20Pediatric%20Mental%20Health%20-%20A%20Study%20of%20Private%20Healthcare%20Claims%20-%20A%20FAIR%20Health%20White%20Paper.pdf

Healthcare Financial Management Association. (2020, October 7). *Major insurers roll back no-cost sharing telehealth services.* HFMA. https://www.hfma.org/topics/technology/article/-major-insurers-roll-back-no-cost-sharing-telehealth-services.html

Hirko, K. A., Kerver, J. M., Ford, S., Szafranski, C., Beckett, J., Kitchen, C., & Wendling, A. L. (2020). Telehealth in response to the COVID-19 pandemic: Implications for rural health disparities. [Retrieved from https://doi.org/10.1093/jamia/ocaa156]. *Journal of the American Medical Informatics Association, 27*(11), 1816–1818.

Hobbes, T. (1651). *Leviathan or The Matter, Forme and Power of a Commonwealth Ecclesiasticall and Civil.* Academic Press.

Hollander, J., & Carr, B. (2020). Virtually Perfect?? Telemedicine for COVID-19. *New England Journal of Medicine, 382*https://doi.org/10.1056/NEJMp2003539 doi:.

HUD (US Department of Housing and Urban Development). (2020). Housing Choice Vouchers Fact Sheet. [Data set]. https://www.hud.gov/topics/housing_choice_voucher_program_section_8.

Hwang, C. J., & Lappan, C. M. (2014). Utilization of Telemedicine in the U.S. Military in a Deployed Setting. *Military Medicine, 179*, 1347–1353.

IMF, World Economic Outlook, Washington, DC: IMF, various issues.

INS (United States Department of Justice Immigration and Naturalization Service). (1999). Proposed Rule on Inadmissibility and Deportability on Public Charge Grounds; Field Guidance on Deportability and Inadmissibility on Public Charge Grounds; Proposed Rule and Notice. *Federal Register, 64*(101).

Interstate Medical Licensure Compact. (2020). *A Faster Pathway to Physician Licensure.* IMLCC. https://www.imlcc.org/

Jansson, B. S. (2001). The Reluctant Welfare State: American Social Welfare Policies-Past, Present, and Future (4th ed., pp. 194, 199). Wadsworth/Thomson Learning.

Journal, H. I. P. A. A. (2014-2020). *What is the HITECH Act*. Retrieved November 29, 2020, from https://www.hipaajournal.com/what-is-the-hitech-act/

Journal, H. I. P. A. A. (2018). *What is the HITECH Act?* Retrieved November 29, 2020, from https://www.hipaajournal.com/what-is-the-hitech-act/

Kandel, W. (2021). The Trump Administration's "Zero Tolerance" Immigration Enforcement Policy. *Congressional Research Service R45266*. https://sgp.fas.org/crs/homesec/R45266.pdf

Kaplan, M. (1995). Teoría y realidad del Estado en América Latina. In M. Mols and J. Thesings (eds.), El Estado en América Latina. Fundación Konrad Adenauer.

Karagiannis, N., & Madjd-Sadjadi, Z. (2007). *Modern State Intervention in the Era of Globalisation*. Edward Elgar.

Keynes, J. M. (1940). *How to Pay for the War: A Radical Plan for the Chancellor of the Exchequer*. Macmillan.

Lee, M. (2020). Coronavirus fears show how 'model minority' Asian Americans become the 'yellow peril. *NBC News, Self-Explanatory blog*. https://www.nbcnews.com/think/opinion/coronavirus-fears-show-how-model-minority-asian-americans-become-yellow-ncna1151671 .

Lefkovitz, N. (2021, January 14). *Happy First Birthday, NIST Privacy Framework!* NIST. https://www.nist.gov/blogs/cybersecurity-insights/happy-first-birthday-nist-privacy-framework

Lerner, A. P. (1943, February). Functional Finance and the Federal Debt. *Social Research, 10*(1), 38–51.

Li, R., Sen Pei, B. C., Song, Y., Zhang, T., Yang, W., & Shaman, J. (2020). Substantial undocumented infection facilitates the rapid dissemination of novel coronavirus (SARS-CoV2). *Science Magazine*. http://science.sciencemag.org/content/early/2020/03/13/science.abb3221.abstract

Maheu, M., & Whitten, P. Allen, & Ace. (2002). E-Health, Telehealth, and Telemedicine: A Guide to Startup and Success. John Wiley & Sons.

Márquez, G. G. (1988). Love in the Time of Cholera. 1st American ed., Edith Grossman, trans. New York: Alfred A. Knopf.

Marx, J. D. (1997). Federated Fundraising. In *The International Encyclopedia of Public Policy and Administration* (Vol. 2, pp. 877–881). Westview Press.

Mathematica. (2020, November 23). *Maintaining Flexible Telehealth Policies After COVID-19*. Retrieved November 25, 2020, from https://www.mathematica.org/our-publications-and-findings/publications/maintaining-flexible-telehealth-policies-after-covid-19

Mayo Clinic. (2020). *Managing your health in the age of Wi-Fi*. Retrieved November 29, 2020, from https://www.mayoclinic.org/healthy-lifestyle/consumer-health/in-depth/telehealth/art-20044878

Mayo Clinic. (2020, May 15). *Telehealth: Technology meets health care.* Retrieved November 28, 2020, from https://www.mayoclinic.org/healthy-lifestyle/consumer-health/in-depth/telehealth/art-20044878

McFadyen, J. (2020) Immigrants and Public Benefits. *ThoughtCo.* https://www.thoughtco.com/immigrants-and-public-benefits-1951828.

Medical Justice. (2016, August 12). *Liability in Telemedicine: "Can you sue me now?".* Retrieved March 15, 2021, from https://medicaljustice.com/liability-telemedicine-can-sue-now/

Medicare.gov. (2021). *Telehealth.* Medicare. https://www.medicare.gov/coverage/telehealth

Moley, R. (1966). *The First New Deal.* Harcourt, Brace & World, Inc.

Nagata, J. M. (2020). Rapid Scale-Up of Telehealth During the COVID-19 Pandemicand Implications for Subspecialty Care in Rural Areas. *The Journal of Rural Health.* doi:10.1111/jrh.12433

National Institute of Standards and Technology. (2020, January 16). *NIST Privacy Framework: A Tool for Improving Privacy Through Enterprise Risk Management, Version 1.0.* NIST. https://nvlpubs.nist.gov/nistpubs/CSWP/NIST.CSWP.01162020.pdf

National Rural Health Association. (2017, February). A Rural-Urban Comparison of Hospitals Participating in the Medicare Electronic Health Record Incentive Program. *Rural Health.* https://www.ruralhealthweb.org/NRHA/media/Emerge_NRHA/Advocacy/Policy%20documents/Medicare-Electronic-Health_Feb-2017_NRHA-Policy-Paper.pdf

NEJM Catalyst. (2018, February 1). Innovations in Care Delivery. *New England Journal of Medicine.* https://catalyst.nejm.org/doi/full/10.1056/CAT.18.0268

New York State Department of Health. (2021). *Foreign Countries with Universal Health Care.* NYSDH. https://www.health.ny.gov/regulations/hcra/univ_hlth_care.htm

Nguyen, C. M. (2020). Reduction in Medical Evacuations from Iraq and Syria Following Introduction of an Asynchronous Telehealth System. *Military Medicine, 185*(9-10), 1693–1699.

Nicholas James Rademacher, M. G. (2019). Use of Telemedicine to Screen Patients in the Emergency Department: Matched Cohort Study Evaluating Efficiency and Patient Safety of Telemedicine. *JMIR Medical Informatics, 7*(2).

NLIHC (National Low Income Housing Coalition). (2020). President Trump Proposes Drastic Cuts to Affordable Housing Programs. *Analysis of President Trump's FY2020 Budget Request.* https://nlihc.org/resource/analysis-president-trumps-fy2020-budget-request

Novak, M. (2012, March 14). Telemedicine Predicted in 1925. *Smithsonian Magazine.* https://www.smithsonianmag.com/history/telemedicine-predicted-in-1925-124140942/

Novara, G. C. (2020). Telehealth in Urology: A systematic review of the literature. How much can telemedicine be useful during and after the Covid-19 Pandemic? *European Urology.*

Nuzzo, J. (2019). Responding to a Mumps Outbreak in a Hard-to-Reach Community. In *Outbreak Observatory Report*. John's Hopkins Bloomberg School of Public Health. https://www.outbreakobservatory.org/outbreakthursday-1/10/10/2019/responding-to-a-mumps-outbreak-in-a-hard-to-reach-community.

Obinger, H., & Schmitt, K. (2018, May). The Impact of the Second World War on Postwar Social Spending. *European Journal of Political Research*, *57*(2), 496–517. doi:10.1111/1475-6765.12236

OECD, (n.d.). *National Accounts,* (vol. II). OECD. https://www.oecd-ilibrary.org/economics/national-accounts-of-oecd-countries-volume-ii-detailed-tables_19961995

Office for Civil Rights. (2013, January 25). Modifications to the HIPAA Privacy, Security, Enforcement, and Breach Notification Rules Under the Health Information Technology for Economic and Clinical Health Act and the Genetic Information Nondiscrimination Act; Other Modifications to the HIPAA Rules. *Department of Health and Human Services,* p. 5634. https://www.federalregister.gov/documents/2013/01/25/2013-01073/modifications-to-the-hipaa-privacy-security-enforcement-and-breach-notification-rules-under-the

Office of the National Coordinator for Health Information Technology. (2016, November). *Federal Telehealth Compendium.* Federal Office of Rural Health Policy. https://mtelehealth.com/wp-content/uploads/2019/10/Federal-Telehealth-Compendium.pdf

Ohannessian, R., Duong, T., & Odone, A. (2020). Global Telemedicine Implementation and Integration Within Health Systems to Fight the COVID-19 Pandemic: A Call to Action. *JMIR Public Health and Surveillannce, 6*(2).

Palley, T. I. (1998, Fall). The Economics of Social Security: An Old Keynesian Perspective. *Journal of Post Keynesian Economics*, *21*(1), 94. doi:10.1080/01603477.1998.11490181

Poe, K. (2000). Telemedicine Liability: Texas and Other States Delve into the Uncertainties of Health Care Delivery via Advanced Communications Technology. *Review of Litigation*, *20*(3), 681–708. https://heinonline.org/HOL/P?h=hein.journals/rol20&i=699

Polychroniou, C. J. (2021). So-called Democratic 'Moderates' Are Actually Right-wingers Who Have Always Thrown up Roadblocks to Social Progress. *Common Dreams*. https://www.commondreams.org/views/2021/09/14/so-called-democratic-moderates-are-actually-right-wingers-who-have-always-thrown

Post, J. E., Lawrence, A. T., & Weber, J. (2002). *Business And Society: Corporate Strategy, Public Policy, Ethics* (10th ed.). McGraw-Hill.

Relman, A. (1980). The New Medical-Industrial Complex. *The New England Journal of Medicine*, 303.

Relman, A. (2007). *A Second Opition: Rescuing American's Health Care*. Public Affairs.

Rizzi, A. M. (2020, September 16). The new 'normal': Rapid adoption of telemedicine in orthopaedics during the COVID-19 pandemic. *Injury*.

Robinson, S., Varhol, R., Ramamurthy, V., Denehy, M., Hendrie, D., O'Leary, P., & Selvey, L. (2015). The Australian primary healthcare experiment: A national survey of Medicare Locals. *BMJ Open*, *5*(3), e007191. doi:10.1136/bmjopen-2014-007191 PMID:25818276

Schteingart, M. (1999). *Políticas Sociales para los Pobres en América Latina*. Miguel Ángel Porrúa.

Scriven, D. (2015). Tuskegee & Obamacare: Fulfilling America's Promise of Health Care Justice. Journal of Healthcare, Science, and the Humanities, 5(2), 113-123.

Sen, Amartya. (2003). La economía política de la focalización. *Comercio Exterior, 53*(6).

Shiferaw, F., & Zolfo, M. (2012, April 2). The role of information communication technology (ICT) towards universal health coverage: the first steps of a telemedicine project in Ethiopia. *Global Health Action, 5*. https://www.ncbi.nlm.nih.gov/pmc/articles/PMC3318899/

Simons, M. (1988). García Márquez on Love, Plagues and Politics. *The New York Times*.

Simpson, A. T., Doarn, C. R., & Garber, S. J. (2020). Interagency Cooperation in the Twilight of the Great Society: Telemedicine, NASA, and the Papago Nation. *Journal of Policy History*, *32*(1), 25–51. doi:10.1017/S0898030619000265

Skocpol, T. (1995). Protecting Soldiers and Mothers: The Political Origins Of Social Policy. In *The United States* (pp. 290–293). Harvard University.

Social Programs in the United States. (n.d.). In *Wikipedia*. https://en.wikipedia.org/wiki/Social_programs_in_the_United_States

Stein, M. M. (2020, 03 11). *Coronavirus Funding Package Waives Medicare Telehealth Restrictions*. Winston-Salem State University. https://search-proquest-com.courseinfo.wssu.edu/docview/2375735192?pq-origsite=summon

Straube, B. M. (2013). A Role for Government: An Observation on Federal Healthcare Efforts in Prevention. *American Journal of Preventive Medicine*, *44*(1), S39–S42. doi:10.1016/j.amepre.2012.09.009 PMID:23195165

Tax Policy Center. (2021). *What Are the Sources of Revenue for the Federal Government*. Urban Institute and Brookings Institution. https://www.taxpolicycenter.org/briefing-book/what-are-sources-revenue-federal-government

TeleHealth Access for Seniors. (n.d.). *TeleHealth Access*. TeleHealth Access for Seniors. https://www.telehealthforseniors.org/

The Evolving Enterprise. (2020, April 24). *Telemedicine search queries jump by 525%, Ethiopia ranks highest*. The Evolving Enterprise. https://www.theee.ai/2020/04/24/2038-telemedicine-search-queries-jump-by-525-ethiopia-ranks-highest/

The Office of the National Coordinator for Health Information Technology (ONC). (2019, October 17). *What is telehealth? How is telehealth different from telemedicine?* HRSA. https://www.healthit.gov/faq/what-telehealth-how-telehealth-different-telemedicine

Totten, A., Hansen, R., Wagner, J., Stillman, L., Ivlev, I., Davis-O'Reilly, C., & McDonagh, M. (2019). Telehealth for Acute and Chronic Care Consultations. *Europe PMC.* https://europepmc.org/article/NBK/nbk547239

Trattner, W. I. (1999). From Poor Law To Welfare State: A History Of Social Welfare. In *America* (6th ed., p. 348). The Free Press.

U.S. Department of Health and Human Services. (2020, May 07). *HIPAA flexibility during DOVID-19.* HHS. https://www.hhs.gov/coronavirus/telehealth/index.html

U.S. Department of Veterans Affairs. (2020). *Office of Rural Health.* DVA. https://www.ruralhealth.va.gov/aboutus/programs.asp

U.S. Health Resources & Services Administration. (2017). *About HRSA.* HRSA. https://www.hrsa.gov/about/index.htm

U.S. Health Resources & Services Administration. (2017). *Federal Office of Rural Health Policy.* HRSA. https://www.hrsa.gov/rural-health/index.html

U.S. Health Resources & Services Administration. (2017). *Telehealth Programs.* HRSA. https://www.hrsa.gov/rural-health/telehealth

UN (United Nations). (2003). The Challenge of Slums. In *United Nations Human Settlements Program 2003 Global Report on Human Settlements. London and Sterling*. Earthscan Publications.

UNC School of Medicine. (2020, January 2). *The Ultimate Telemedicine: UNC Expert Helps Treat Astronaut's Blood Clot During NASA Mission.* Retrieved November 29, 2020, from https://news.unchealthcare.org/2020/01/telemedicine-astronauts-blood-clot-nasa/

UNDP. (United Nations Development Program) (1999). Human Development Report. Oxford University Press.

USCIS (United States Citizenship and Immigration Services). (2020). Public Charge Fact Sheet. https://www.uscis.gov/news/fact-sheets/public-charge-fact-sheet .

Valinsky, J. (2020). Estas 14 compañías han crecido durante la pandemia de coronavirus. *CNN Espanol.* https://cnnespanol.cnn.com/2020/05/07/estas-14-companias-han-crecido-durante-la-pandemia-de-coronavirus/

Wade, R. H. (2014). The Developmental State: New Perspectives. JICA/IPD Task Force Meeting on Industrial Policy & Transformation, Jordan, June 5-6.

Wallut, L., Peyron, C., Hervieu-Bègue, M., Osseby, G.-V., Giroud, M., Legris, N., ... Lejeune, C. (2020, April). Efficiency of telemedicine for acute stroke: A cost-effectiveness analysis from a French pilot study. *International Journal of Technology Assessment in Health Care, 36*(2), 126–132.

Weisbrot, M. (2019). Puerto Rico's Botched Disaster Relief, Unsustainable Debt, and Economic Failure Linked to its Colonial Status. In *CEPR article, May 30*. Center for Economic and Policy Research. https://www.cepr.net/puerto-rico-s-botched-disaster-relief-unsustainable-debt-and-economic-failure-linked-to-its-colonial-status/

Wicklund, E. (2020, December 2). CMS Finalizes Telehealth, RPM Coverage in 2021 Physician Fee Schedule. *mHealth Intelligence*. https://mhealthintelligence.com/news/cms-finalizes-telehealth-rpm-coverage-in-2021-physician-fee-schedule

Wicklund, E. (2020, January 2). NASA Uses Telehealth to Answer a Space Station Medical Emergency. *mHealth Intelligence*. https://mhealthintelligence.com/news/nasa-uses-telehealth-to-answer-a-space-station-medical-emergency

Wicklund, E. (2021, March 29). New Bills Target Telehealth Coverage for Substance Abuse, Mental Health Services. *mHealth Intelligence*. https://mhealthintelligence.com/news/new-bills-target-telehealth-coverage-for-substance-abuse-mental-health-services

Wong, M. Y., Gunasekeran, D. V., Nusinovici, S., Sabanayagam, C., Yeo, K. K., Cheng, C.-Y., & Tham, Y.-C. (2021). Telehealth Demand Trends During the COVID-19 Pandemic in the Top 50 Most Affected Countries: Infodemiological Evaluation. *JMIR Public Health and Surveillance*, *7*(2).

World Health Organization. (2016). *Telehealth: Analysis of third global survey on eHeallth based on the reported data by countries, 2016*. WHO. https://www.who.int/gho/goe/telehealth/en/

Wray, L. R. (2005). Social Security's 70th Anniversary: Surviving 20 Years of Reform. In *Policy Note 2005/6. Annandale-on-Hudson*. Levy Economics Institute of Bard College.

Related References

To continue our tradition of advancing information science and technology research, we have compiled a list of recommended IGI Global readings. These references will provide additional information and guidance to further enrich your knowledge and assist you with your own research and future publications.

Abdel-Hameid, S. O., & Wilson, E. (2018). Gender, Organization, and Change in Sudan. In N. Mahtab, T. Haque, I. Khan, M. Islam, & I. Wahid (Eds.), *Handbook of Research on Women's Issues and Rights in the Developing World* (pp. 107–120). Hershey, PA: IGI Global. doi:10.4018/978-1-5225-3018-3.ch007

Abdullahi, R. B. (2018). Volunteerism in Urban Development the Case of Non-Cash, Non-Digital Crowdfunding Growth in Nigeria. In U. Benna & A. Benna (Eds.), *Crowdfunding and Sustainable Urban Development in Emerging Economies* (pp. 188–210). Hershey, PA: IGI Global. doi:10.4018/978-1-5225-3952-0.ch010

Abioye, T. O., Oyesomi, K., Ajiboye, E., Omidiora, S., & Oyero, O. (2017). Education, Gender, and Child-Rights: Salient Issues in SDGS Years in ADO-ODO/OTA Local Government Area of Ogun State, Nigeria. In O. Nelson, B. Ojebuyi, & A. Salawu (Eds.), *Impacts of the Media on African Socio-Economic Development* (pp. 141–154). Hershey, PA: IGI Global. doi:10.4018/978-1-5225-1859-4.ch009

Adalı, G. K. (2022). Measuring the Attitudes of Governmental Policies and the Public Towards the COVID-19 Pandemic. In Ş. Omeraki Çekirdekci, Ö. İngün Karkış, & S. Gönültaş (Eds.), *Handbook of Research on Interdisciplinary Perspectives on the Threats and Impacts of Pandemics* (pp. 163–187). IGI Global. https://doi.org/10.4018/978-1-7998-8674-7.ch009

Adisa, W. B. (2018). Land Use Policy and Urban Sprawl in Nigeria: Land Use and the Emergence of Urban Sprawl. In A. Eneanya (Ed.), *Handbook of Research on Environmental Policies for Emergency Management and Public Safety* (pp. 256–274). Hershey, PA: IGI Global. doi:10.4018/978-1-5225-3194-4.ch014

Afolabi, O. S., Amao-Kolawole, T. G., Shittu, A. K., & Oguntokun, O. O. (2018). Rule of Law, Governance, and Sustainable Development: The Nigerian Perspective. In K. Teshager Alemu & M. Abebe Alebachew (Eds.), *Handbook of Research on Sustainable Development and Governance Strategies for Economic Growth in Africa* (pp. 273–290). Hershey, PA: IGI Global. doi:10.4018/978-1-5225-3247-7.ch015

Agyemang, O. S. (2018). Institutional Structures and the Prevalence of Foreign Ownership of Firms: Empirical Evidence From Africa. In K. Teshager Alemu & M. Abebe Alebachew (Eds.), *Handbook of Research on Sustainable Development and Governance Strategies for Economic Growth in Africa* (pp. 455–479). Hershey, PA: IGI Global. doi:10.4018/978-1-5225-3247-7.ch024

Aham-Anyanwu, N. M., & Li, H. (2017). E-State: Realistic or Utopian? *International Journal of Public Administration in the Digital Age*, *4*(2), 56–76. doi:10.4018/IJPADA.2017040105

Al Balushi, T., & Ali, S. (2020). Theoretical Approach for Instrument Development in Measuring User-Perceived E-Government Service Quality: A Case of Oman E-Government Services. *International Journal of Electronic Government Research*, *16*(1), 40–58. doi:10.4018/IJEGR.2020010103

Al-Jamal, M., & Abu-Shanab, E. (2018). Open Government: The Line between Privacy and Transparency. *International Journal of Public Administration in the Digital Age*, *5*(2), 64–75. doi:10.4018/IJPADA.2018040106

Alsaç, U. (2017). EKAP: Turkey's Centralized E-Procurement System. In R. Shakya (Ed.), *Digital Governance and E-Government Principles Applied to Public Procurement* (pp. 126–150). Hershey, PA: IGI Global. doi:10.4018/978-1-5225-2203-4.ch006

Amadi, L. A., & Igwe, P. (2018). Open Government and Bureaucratic Secrecy in the Developing Democracies: Africa in Perspective. In A. Kok (Ed.), *Proliferation of Open Government Initiatives and Systems* (pp. 1–28). Hershey, PA: IGI Global. doi:10.4018/978-1-5225-4987-1.ch001

Arble, E., & Arnetz, B. B. (2021). Four Fundamental Principles to Enhance Police Performance and Community Safety. In E. Arble & B. Arnetz (Eds.), *Interventions, Training, and Technologies for Improved Police Well-Being and Performance* (pp. 231–245). IGI Global. https://doi.org/10.4018/978-1-7998-6820-0.ch015

Arora, G. C. (2020). The Problem of Climate-Induced Displacement: Analyzing the International Framework on Protection of Rights of Climate Migrants. In R. Das & N. Mandal (Eds.), *Interdisciplinary Approaches to Public Policy and Sustainability* (pp. 67–82). IGI Global. https://doi.org/10.4018/978-1-7998-0315-7.ch004

Arora, T., & Mehra, N. (2021). Administration of Civil Justice in India: Ancient and Modern Perspectives. In E. Yin & N. Kofie (Eds.), *Advancing Civil Justice Reform and Conflict Resolution in Africa and Asia: Comparative Analyses and Case Studies* (pp. 17–45). IGI Global. https://doi.org/10.4018/978-1-7998-7898-8.ch002

Arteta, A. (2019). *Democracy and Government: Making Decisions*. IGI Global. doi:10.4018/978-1-5225-7558-0.ch001

Asante, M., & Botchway, T. P. (2021). Shielding Members of Parliament Against Court Summons: Interrogating the Question of Parliamentary Immunity. In E. Yin & N. Kofie (Eds.), *Advancing Civil Justice Reform and Conflict Resolution in Africa and Asia: Comparative Analyses and Case Studies* (pp. 210–229). IGI Global. https://doi.org/10.4018/978-1-7998-7898-8.ch012

Ateş, V. (2021). Critical Antecedents of Trust in E-Government Services in Turkey. In C. Babaoğlu, E. Akman, & O. Kulaç (Eds.), *Handbook of Research on Global Challenges for Improving Public Services and Government Operations* (pp. 94–116). IGI Global. https://doi.org/10.4018/978-1-7998-4978-0.ch006

Ayeni, A. O. (2018). Environmental Policies for Emergency Management and Public Safety: Implementing Green Policy and Community Participation. In A. Eneanya (Ed.), *Handbook of Research on Environmental Policies for Emergency Management and Public Safety* (pp. 40–59). Hershey, PA: IGI Global. doi:10.4018/978-1-5225-3194-4.ch003

Ayodele, J. O. (2017). The Influence of Migration and Crime on Development in Lagos, Nigeria. In G. Afolayan & A. Akinwale (Eds.), *Global Perspectives on Development Administration and Cultural Change* (pp. 192–230). Hershey, PA: IGI Global. doi:10.4018/978-1-5225-0629-4.ch009

Baarda, R. (2017). Digital Democracy in Authoritarian Russia: Opportunity for Participation, or Site of Kremlin Control? In R. Luppicini & R. Baarda (Eds.), *Digital Media Integration for Participatory Democracy* (pp. 87–100). Hershey, PA: IGI Global. doi:10.4018/978-1-5225-2463-2.ch005

Balakrishnan, K. (2017). The Rationale for Offsets in Defence Acquisition from a Theoretical Perspective. In K. Burgess & P. Antill (Eds.), *Emerging Strategies in Defense Acquisitions and Military Procurement* (pp. 263–276). Hershey, PA: IGI Global. doi:10.4018/978-1-5225-0599-0.ch015

Banerjee, S. (2017). Globalization and Human Rights: How Globalization Can Be a Tool to Protect the Human Rights. In C. Akrivopoulou (Ed.), *Defending Human Rights and Democracy in the Era of Globalization* (pp. 1–16). Hershey, PA: IGI Global. doi:10.4018/978-1-5225-0723-9.ch001

Bessant, J. (2017). Digital Humour, Gag Laws, and the Liberal Security State. In R. Luppicini & R. Baarda (Eds.), *Digital Media Integration for Participatory Democracy* (pp. 204–221). Hershey, PA: IGI Global. doi:10.4018/978-1-5225-2463-2.ch010

Bhat, M. Y. (2020). Environmental Problems of Delhi and Governmental Concern. In M. Merviö (Ed.), *Global Issues and Innovative Solutions in Healthcare, Culture, and the Environment* (pp. 133–167). IGI Global. https://doi.org/10.4018/978-1-7998-3576-9.ch008

Bhat, R. A. (2021). Identification of Various Dimensions and Indicators of Immigrant Integration Into Global Scenarios. In M. Mafukata (Ed.), *Impact of Immigration and Xenophobia on Development in Africa* (pp. 247–260). IGI Global. https://doi.org/10.4018/978-1-7998-7099-9.ch014

Boachie, C. (2017). Public Financial Management and Systems of Accountability in Sub-National Governance in Developing Economies. In E. Schoburgh & R. Ryan (Eds.), *Handbook of Research on Sub-National Governance and Development* (pp. 193–217). Hershey, PA: IGI Global. doi:10.4018/978-1-5225-1645-3.ch009

Boachie, C., & Adu-Darko, E. (2018). Socio-Economic Impact of Foreign Direct Investment in Developing Countries. In V. Malepati & C. Gowri (Eds.), *Foreign Direct Investments (FDIs) and Opportunities for Developing Economies in the World Market* (pp. 66–81). Hershey, PA: IGI Global. doi:10.4018/978-1-5225-3026-8.ch004

Bogdanoski, M., Stoilkovski, M., & Risteski, A. (2020). Novel First Responder Digital Forensics Tool as a Support to Law Enforcement. In I. Management Association (Ed.), *Improving the Safety and Efficiency of Emergency Services: Emerging Tools and Technologies for First Responders* (pp. 239-270). IGI Global. https://doi.org/10.4018/978-1-7998-2535-7.ch011

Borràs, S. (2017). Rights of Nature to Protect Human Rights in Times of Environmental Crisis. In C. Akrivopoulou (Ed.), *Defending Human Rights and Democracy in the Era of Globalization* (pp. 225–261). Hershey, PA: IGI Global. doi:10.4018/978-1-5225-0723-9.ch010

Bouaziz, F. (2021). E-Government and Digital Transformation: A Conceptual Framework for Risk Factors Identification. In K. Sandhu (Ed.), *Disruptive Technology and Digital Transformation for Business and Government* (pp. 67–90). IGI Global. https://doi.org/10.4018/978-1-7998-8583-2.ch004

Bradford, A. C., McElroy, H. K., & Rosenblatt, R. (2019). Social Climate Change and the Modern Police Department: Millennials, Marijuana, and Mass Media. In I. Management Association (Ed.), *Police Science: Breakthroughs in Research and Practice* (pp. 34-51). IGI Global. https://doi.org/10.4018/978-1-5225-7672-3.ch003

Brusca, I., Olmo, J., & Labrador, M. (2018). Characterizing the Risk Factors for Financial Sustainability in Spanish Local Governments. In M. Rodríguez Bolívar & M. López Subires (Eds.), *Financial Sustainability and Intergenerational Equity in Local Governments* (pp. 206–223). Hershey, PA: IGI Global. doi:10.4018/978-1-5225-3713-7.ch009

Budd, J. R., & Littrell, M. W. (2021). Law Enforcement Challenges to Gathering Intelligence in the Street: The Fourth Amendment. In E. de Silva & A. Abeyagoonesekera (Eds.), *Intelligence and Law Enforcement in the 21st Century* (pp. 18–40). IGI Global. https://doi.org/10.4018/978-1-7998-7904-6.ch002

Bush, C. L. (2021). Policing Strategies and Approaches to Improving Community Relations: Black Citizens' Perceptions of Law Enforcement Efforts to Intentionally Strengthen Relationships. In M. Pittaro (Ed.), *Global Perspectives on Reforming the Criminal Justice System* (pp. 56–75). IGI Global. https://doi.org/10.4018/978-1-7998-6884-2.ch004

Canto Moniz, G. (2020). Is There Anything Left of the Portuguese Law Implementing the GDPR?: The Decision of the Portuguese Supervisory Authority. In M. Tzanou (Ed.), *Personal Data Protection and Legal Developments in the European Union* (pp. 125–139). IGI Global. https://doi.org/10.4018/978-1-5225-9489-5.ch007

Casoria, M., & AlSarraf, E. M. (2020). The Impact of the GDPR on Extra-EU Legal Systems: The Case of the Kingdom of Bahrain. In M. Tzanou (Ed.), *Personal Data Protection and Legal Developments in the European Union* (pp. 224–237). IGI Global. https://doi.org/10.4018/978-1-5225-9489-5.ch011

Chaves, A. (2022). Government Response Capacity to the COVID-19 Pandemic: Estimating the Impact of Lockdown Measures in Colombia. In G. Antošová (Ed.), *Innovative Strategic Planning and International Collaboration for the Mitigation of Global Crises* (pp. 114–137). IGI Global. https://doi.org/10.4018/978-1-7998-8339-5.ch008

Chen, M., & Su, F. (2017). Global Civic Engagement as an Empowering Device for Cross-Ethnic and Cross-Cultural Understanding in Taiwan. In R. Shin (Ed.), *Convergence of Contemporary Art, Visual Culture, and Global Civic Engagement* (pp. 24–45). Hershey, PA: IGI Global. doi:10.4018/978-1-5225-1665-1.ch002

Chigwata, T. C. (2017). Fiscal Decentralization: Constraints to Revenue-Raising by Local Government in Zimbabwe. In E. Schoburgh & R. Ryan (Eds.), *Handbook of Research on Sub-National Governance and Development* (pp. 218–240). Hershey, PA: IGI Global. doi:10.4018/978-1-5225-1645-3.ch010

Chowdhury, M. A. (2017). The Nexus Between Institutional Quality and Foreign Direct Investments (FDI) in South Asia: Dynamic Heterogeneous Panel Approach. In T. Dorożyński & A. Kuna-Marszałek (Eds.), *Outward Foreign Direct Investment (FDI) in Emerging Market Economies* (pp. 293–310). Hershey, PA: IGI Global. doi:10.4018/978-1-5225-2345-1.ch015

Christopher, M. E., & Tsushima, V. G. (2017). Police Interactions with Persons-in-Crisis: Emergency Psychological Services and Jail Diversion. In C. Mitchell & E. Dorian (Eds.), *Police Psychology and Its Growing Impact on Modern Law Enforcement* (pp. 274–294). Hershey, PA: IGI Global. doi:10.4018/978-1-5225-0813-7.ch014

Ciftci, D. (2022). Digital Citizenship and E-Government Integration: The Case of North Cyprus. In E. Öngün, N. Pembecioğlu, & U. Gündüz (Eds.), *Handbook of Research on Digital Citizenship and Management During Crises* (pp. 34–55). IGI Global. https://doi.org/10.4018/978-1-7998-8421-7.ch003

Citro, F., Lucianelli, G., & Santis, S. (2018). Financial Conditions, Financial Sustainability, and Intergenerational Equity in Local Governments: A Literature Review. In M. Rodríguez Bolívar & M. López Subires (Eds.), *Financial Sustainability and Intergenerational Equity in Local Governments* (pp. 101–124). Hershey, PA: IGI Global. doi:10.4018/978-1-5225-3713-7.ch005

Correa de Mello, M. B. (2019). The Information Access Law as a Full Constitutional Citizenship Instrument. In A. Melro & L. Oliveira (Eds.), *Constitutional Knowledge and Its Impact on Citizenship Exercise in a Networked Society* (pp. 55–72). IGI Global. https://doi.org/10.4018/978-1-5225-8350-9.ch003

Covell, C. E. (2018). Theoretical Application of Public Sector Planning and Budgeting. In M. Rodríguez Bolívar & M. López Subires (Eds.), *Financial Sustainability and Intergenerational Equity in Local Governments* (pp. 248–279). Hershey, PA: IGI Global. doi:10.4018/978-1-5225-3713-7.ch011

Cunha, A. M., Ferreira, A. D., & Fernandes, M. J. (2018). The Impact of Accounting Information and Socioeconomic Factors in the Re-Election of Portuguese Mayors. In G. Azevedo, J. da Silva Oliveira, R. Marques, & A. Ferreira (Eds.), *Handbook of Research on Modernization and Accountability in Public Sector Management* (pp. 406–432). Hershey, PA: IGI Global. doi:10.4018/978-1-5225-3731-1.ch019 da Rosa, I., & de Almeida, J. (2017). Digital Transformation in the Public Sector: Electronic Procurement in Portugal. In R. Shakya (Ed.), *Digital Governance and E-Government Principles Applied to Public Procurement* (pp. 99–125). Hershey, PA: IGI Global. doi:10.4018/978-1-5225-2203-4.ch005

Daramola, O. (2018). Revisiting the Legal Framework of Urban Planning in the Global South: An Explanatory Example of Nigeria. In K. Teshager Alemu & M. Abebe Alebachew (Eds.), *Handbook of Research on Sustainable Development and Governance Strategies for Economic Growth in Africa* (pp. 258–271). Hershey, PA: IGI Global. doi:10.4018/978-1-5225-3247-7.ch014

Dau, L. A., Moore, E. M., Soto, M. A., & LeBlanc, C. R. (2017). How Globalization Sparked Entrepreneurship in the Developing World: The Impact of Formal Economic and Political Linkages. In B. Christiansen & F. Kasarcı (Eds.), *Corporate Espionage, Geopolitics, and Diplomacy Issues in International Business* (pp. 72–91). Hershey, PA: IGI Global. doi:10.4018/978-1-5225-1031-4.ch005

De Man, P. (2019). In-Situ Resource Utilization: Legal Aspects. In A. Nakarada Pecujlic & M. Tugnoli (Eds.), *Promoting Productive Cooperation Between Space Lawyers and Engineers* (pp. 211–224). IGI Global. https://doi.org/10.4018/978-1-5225-7256-5.ch013

Drenner, K. (2017). Introduction to Faith in State Legislatures: Land of the Brave and the Home of the Free – The Star-Spangled Banner. In *Impacts of Faith-Based Decision Making on the Individual-Level Legislative Process: Emerging Research and Opportunities* (pp. 1–25). Hershey, PA: IGI Global. doi:10.4018/978-1-5225-2388-8.ch001

Drenner, K. (2017). The Holy Wars of Marriage. In *Impacts of Faith-Based Decision Making on the Individual-Level Legislative Process: Emerging Research and Opportunities* (pp. 92–116). Hershey, PA: IGI Global. doi:10.4018/978-1-5225-2388-8.ch004

Drenner, K. (2017). The Implications of Religious Liberty. In *Impacts of Faith-Based Decision Making on the Individual-Level Legislative Process: Emerging Research and Opportunities* (pp. 143–162). Hershey, PA: IGI Global. doi:10.4018/978-1-5225-2388-8.ch006

Duncan, S. T., & Geczi, H. (2021). Body-Worn Cameras: Panacea or Distraction for Increased Police Use of Force Accountability? In M. Pittaro (Ed.), *Global Perspectives on Reforming the Criminal Justice System* (pp. 1–25). IGI Global. https://doi.org/10.4018/978-1-7998-6884-2.ch001

Duran, D. Ş. (2019). Reflections of the Multi-Level Governance Approach on the Turkish Metropolitan Municipality System: Evaluations on the Metropolitan Law No 6360. In T. Uysal & C. Aldemir (Eds.), *Multi-Level Governance in Developing Economies* (pp. 52–91). IGI Global. https://doi.org/10.4018/978-1-5225-5547-6.ch003

Durnalı, M., & Eriçok, B. (2019). Legal Challenges on Developing Education Policy for Immigrants in Turkey. In I. Management Association (Ed.), *Immigration and Refugee Policy: Breakthroughs in Research and Practice* (pp. 223-237). IGI Global. https://doi.org/10.4018/978-1-5225-8909-9.ch013

Ehalaiye, D., Redmayne, N. B., & Laswad, F. (2020). The Case of Accounting Information for Infrastructural Assets Reporting: Local Government Borrowings and Investment Choices in the Context of Moral Hazard and Local Government Politics. In A. Cunha, A. Ferreira, M. Fernandes, & P. Gomes (Eds.), *Financial Determinants in Local Re-Election Rates: Emerging Research and Opportunities* (pp. 176–201). IGI Global. https://doi.org/10.4018/978-1-5225-7820-8.ch007

Elena, S., & van Schalkwyk, F. (2017). Open Data for Open Justice in Seven Latin American Countries. In C. Jiménez-Gómez & M. Gascó-Hernández (Eds.), *Achieving Open Justice through Citizen Participation and Transparency* (pp. 210–231). Hershey, PA: IGI Global. doi:10.4018/978-1-5225-0717-8.ch011

Eneanya, A. N. (2018). Integrating Ecosystem Management and Environmental Media for Public Policy on Public Health and Safety. In A. Eneanya (Ed.), *Handbook of Research on Environmental Policies for Emergency Management and Public Safety* (pp. 321–338). Hershey, PA: IGI Global. doi:10.4018/978-1-5225-3194-4.ch017

Erickson, G. S. (2019). Sharing Knowledge With the Government: Implications of FOIA Requests. In Y. Albastaki, A. Al-Alawi, & S. Abdulrahman Al-Bassam (Eds.), *Handbook of Research on Implementing Knowledge Management Strategy in the Public Sector* (pp. 143–158). IGI Global. https://doi.org/10.4018/978-1-5225-9639-4.ch007

Essien, E. D. (2018). Strengthening Performance of Civil Society Through Dialogue and Critical Thinking in Nigeria: Its Ethical Implications. In S. Chhabra (Ed.), *Handbook of Research on Civic Engagement and Social Change in Contemporary Society* (pp. 82–102). Hershey, PA: IGI Global. doi:10.4018/978-1-5225-4197-4.ch005

Eweida, A. M. (2021). Urban Laws in Harmony or at Odds With Knowledge-Based Urban Policies: A Case Study on Egypt. In A. Galaby & A. Abdrabo (Eds.), *Handbook of Research on Creative Cities and Advanced Models for Knowledge-Based Urban Development* (pp. 23–40). IGI Global. https://doi.org/10.4018/978-1-7998-4948-3.ch002

Fanaian, T. (2017). The Theocratic Deception Trap: Khomeini's Persuasion Techniques and Communication Patterns in His Books, Guardianship of the Jurist 1979 and Testament 1989. In E. Lewin, E. Bick, & D. Naor (Eds.), *Comparative Perspectives on Civil Religion, Nationalism, and Political Influence* (pp. 62–105). Hershey, PA: IGI Global. doi:10.4018/978-1-5225-0516-7.ch003

Faura-Martínez, U., & Cifuentes-Faura, J. (2020). Does E-Government Promote Transparency and the Fight Against Corruption in the European Union? *International Journal of Electronic Government Research, 16*(4), 42–57. https://doi.org/10.4018/IJEGR.2020100103

Fawsitt, J. (2020). Government Policy and the Disintegration of Village Community Life and Individual Identity in Urbanising Japan. In M. Merviö (Ed.), *Recent Social, Environmental, and Cultural Issues in East Asian Societies* (pp. 76–94). IGI Global. https://doi.org/10.4018/978-1-7998-1807-6.ch005

Fidanoski, F., Sergi, B. S., Simeonovski, K., Naumovski, V., & Sazdovski, I. (2018). Effects of Foreign Capital Entry on the Macedonian Banking Industry: Two-Edged Sword. In B. Sergi, F. Fidanoski, M. Ziolo, & V. Naumovski (Eds.), *Regaining Global Stability After the Financial Crisis* (pp. 308–338). Hershey, PA: IGI Global. doi:10.4018/978-1-5225-4026-7.ch015

Franconi, A. I. (2018). Economic Variations and Their Impact on Labor Legislation Throughout History in Argentina. In S. Amine (Ed.), *Employment Protection Legislation in Emerging Economies* (pp. 77–98). Hershey, PA: IGI Global. doi:10.4018/978-1-5225-4134-9.ch004

Friedrich, P., & Chebotareva, M. (2017). Options for Applying Functional Overlapping Competing Jurisdictions (FOCJs) for Municipal Cooperation in Russia. In M. Lewandowski & B. Kożuch (Eds.), *Public Sector Entrepreneurship and the Integration of Innovative Business Models* (pp. 73–107). Hershey, PA: IGI Global. doi:10.4018/978-1-5225-2215-7.ch004

Garad, A., & Qamari, I. N. (2021). Determining Factors Influencing Establishing E-Service Quality in Developing Countries: A Case Study of Yemen E-Government. *International Journal of Electronic Government Research, 17*(1), 15–30. https://doi.org/10.4018/IJEGR.2021010102

Garita, M. (2018). The Negotiation and Effects of Fiscal Privileges in Guatemala. In M. Garita & C. Bregni (Eds.), *Economic Growth in Latin America and the Impact of the Global Financial Crisis* (pp. 119–137). Hershey, PA: IGI Global. doi:10.4018/978-1-5225-4981-9.ch008

Gascó-Hernández, M. (2017). Digitalizing Police Requirements: Opening up Justice through Collaborative Initiatives. In C. Jiménez-Gómez & M. Gascó-Hernández (Eds.), *Achieving Open Justice through Citizen Participation and Transparency* (pp. 157–172). Hershey, PA: IGI Global. doi:10.4018/978-1-5225-0717-8.ch008

Gáspár-Szilágyi, S. (2017). Human Rights Conditionality in the EU's Newly Concluded Association Agreements with the Eastern Partners. In C. Akrivopoulou (Ed.), *Defending Human Rights and Democracy in the Era of Globalization* (pp. 50–79). Hershey, PA: IGI Global. doi:10.4018/978-1-5225-0723-9.ch003

Gavrielides, T. (2017). Reconciling Restorative Justice with the Law for Violence Against Women in Europe: A Scheme of Structured and Unstructured Models. In D. Halder & K. Jaishankar (Eds.), *Therapeutic Jurisprudence and Overcoming Violence Against Women* (pp. 106–120). Hershey, PA: IGI Global. doi:10.4018/978-1-5225-2472-4.ch007

Gechlik, M., Dai, D., & Beck, J. C. (2017). Open Judiciary in a Closed Society: A Paradox in China? In C. Jiménez-Gómez & M. Gascó-Hernández (Eds.), *Achieving Open Justice through Citizen Participation and Transparency* (pp. 56–92). Hershey, PA: IGI Global. doi:10.4018/978-1-5225-0717-8.ch004

Gerger, A. (2021). Technologies for Connected Government Implementation: Success Factors and Best Practices. In Z. Mahmood (Ed.), *Web 2.0 and Cloud Technologies for Implementing Connected Government* (pp. 36–66). IGI Global. https://doi.org/10.4018/978-1-7998-4570-6.ch003

Germann, S. K. (2019). The International Space Station: Legal Aspects. In A. Nakarada Pecujlic & M. Tugnoli (Eds.), *Promoting Productive Cooperation Between Space Lawyers and Engineers* (pp. 96–113). IGI Global. doi:10.4018/978-1-5225-7256-5.ch007

Gillath, N. (2017). Avoiding Conscription in Israel: Were Women Pawns in the Political Game? In E. Lewin, E. Bick, & D. Naor (Eds.), *Comparative Perspectives on Civil Religion, Nationalism, and Political Influence* (pp. 226–256). Hershey, PA: IGI Global. doi:10.4018/978-1-5225-0516-7.ch009

Górski, J. (2019). Northern Sea Route: International Law Perspectives. In V. Erokhin, T. Gao, & X. Zhang (Eds.), *Handbook of Research on International Collaboration, Economic Development, and Sustainability in the Arctic* (pp. 292–313). IGI Global. https://doi.org/10.4018/978-1-5225-6954-1.ch014

Grant, B., Woods, R., & Tan, S. F. (2017). Subnational Finance in Australia and China: The Case for Municipal Bond Banks. In E. Schoburgh & R. Ryan (Eds.), *Handbook of Research on Sub-National Governance and Development* (pp. 150–166). Hershey, PA: IGI Global. doi:10.4018/978-1-5225-1645-3.ch007

Gurpinar, B. (2018). Supporter, Activist, Rebel, Terrorist: Children in Syria. In C. Akrivopoulou (Ed.), *Global Perspectives on Human Migration, Asylum, and Security* (pp. 97–114). Hershey, PA: IGI Global. doi:10.4018/978-1-5225-2817-3.ch005

Gussen, B. F. (2018). The United States. In *Ranking Economic Performance and Efficiency in the Global Market: Emerging Research and Opportunities* (pp. 109–136). Hershey, PA: IGI Global. doi:10.4018/978-1-5225-2756-5.ch005

Halder, D., & Bhati, D. (2021). Culture, Ethnicity, and Hate Crimes: A Comparative Analysis of Preventive Laws Between India and the USA. In M. Pittaro (Ed.), *Global Perspectives on Reforming the Criminal Justice System* (pp. 236–245). IGI Global. https://doi.org/10.4018/978-1-7998-6884-2.ch013

Haque, T. (2018). Women-Friendly Working Environment in Bangladesh: Critical Analysis. In N. Mahtab, T. Haque, I. Khan, M. Islam, & I. Wahid (Eds.), *Handbook of Research on Women's Issues and Rights in the Developing World* (pp. 52–68). Hershey, PA: IGI Global. doi:10.4018/978-1-5225-3018-3.ch004

Heuva, W. E. (2017). Deferring Citizens' "Right to Know" in an Information Age: The Information Deficit in Namibia. In N. Mhiripiri & T. Chari (Eds.), *Media Law, Ethics, and Policy in the Digital Age* (pp. 245–267). Hershey, PA: IGI Global. doi:10.4018/978-1-5225-2095-5.ch014

Hwangbo, Y. (2022). Government Challenges Over Global Electronic Commerce Using FinTech: Design of Consumer Payment Tax (CPT) System. In M. Anshari, M. Almunawar, & M. Masri (Eds.), *FinTech Development for Financial Inclusiveness* (pp. 197–213). IGI Global. https://doi.org/10.4018/978-1-7998-8447-7.ch011

Ibrahim, F., Suhip, H., Kura, K. M., & Noor, H. M. L. (2022). Exploratory Study on User Satisfaction of E-HRM: Evidence From Brunei Government Employee Management System (GEMS). In P. Ordóñez de Pablos (Eds.), *Handbook of Research on Developing Circular, Digital, and Green Economies in Asia* (pp. 243-271). IGI Global. https://doi.org/10.4018/978-1-7998-8678-5.ch014

Islam, M. R. (2018). Abuse Among Child Domestic Workers in Bangladesh. In I. Tshabangu (Ed.), *Global Ideologies Surrounding Children's Rights and Social Justice* (pp. 1–21). Hershey, PA: IGI Global. doi:10.4018/978-1-5225-2578-3.ch001

Jankovic-Milic, V., & Džunić, M. (2017). Measuring Governance: The Application of Grey Relational Analysis on World Governance Indicators. In J. Stanković, P. Delias, S. Marinković, & S. Rochhia (Eds.), *Tools and Techniques for Economic Decision Analysis* (pp. 104–128). Hershey, PA: IGI Global. doi:10.4018/978-1-5225-0959-2.ch005

Jenkins, B., Semple, T., Quail, J., & Bennell, C. (2021). Optimizing Scenario-Based Training for Law Enforcement. In E. Arble & B. Arnetz (Eds.), *Interventions, Training, and Technologies for Improved Police Well-Being and Performance* (pp. 18–37). IGI Global. https://doi.org/10.4018/978-1-7998-6820-0.ch002

Jiménez-Gómez, C. E. (2017). Open Judiciary Worldwide: Best Practices and Lessons Learnt. In C. Jiménez-Gómez & M. Gascó-Hernández (Eds.), *Achieving Open Justice through Citizen Participation and Transparency* (pp. 1–15). Hershey, PA: IGI Global. doi:10.4018/978-1-5225-0717-8.ch001

Karatzimas, S., & Miquela, C. G. (2018). Two Approaches on Local Governments' Financial Sustainability: Law vs. Practice in Catalan Municipalities. In M. Rodríguez Bolívar & M. López Subires (Eds.), *Financial Sustainability and Intergenerational Equity in Local Governments* (pp. 58–81). Hershey, PA: IGI Global. doi:10.4018/978-1-5225-3713-7.ch003

Khachaturyan, M., & Klicheva, E. (2021). Risks of Introducing E-Governance Into Strategic Management Systems of Russian Companies in the Context of the Pandemic. *International Journal of Electronic Government Research, 17*(4), 84–102. https://doi.org/10.4018/IJEGR.2021100105

Khan, S. A., & Alag, A. (2020). Arbitration in Patent Disputes: To What Extent Is It Possible? In N. Dewani & A. Gurtu (Eds.), *Intellectual Property Rights and the Protection of Traditional Knowledge* (pp. 76–102). IGI Global. https://doi.org/10.4018/978-1-7998-1835-9.ch004

Kirsanov, S., Safonov, E., Tuzcuoglu, F., & Mammadov, Z. (2022). Modern Problems of Staff Training for State and Municipal Services in Russia. In O. Kulaç, C. Babaoğlu, & E. Akman (Eds.), *Public Affairs Education and Training in the 21st Century* (pp. 325–337). IGI Global. https://doi.org/10.4018/978-1-7998-8243-5.ch021

Kita, Y. (2017). An Analysis of a Lay Adjudication System and Open Judiciary: The New Japanese Lay Adjudication System. In C. Jiménez-Gómez & M. Gascó-Hernández (Eds.), *Achieving Open Justice through Citizen Participation and Transparency* (pp. 93–109). Hershey, PA: IGI Global. doi:10.4018/978-1-5225-0717-8.ch005

Kuatova, A., Bekbasarova, T., & Abdrashev, R. (2020). Introducing E-Government in Kazakhstan: The Concept of E-Democracy for the State-Public Interaction. In G. Tazhina & J. Parker (Eds.), *Toward Sustainability Through Digital Technologies and Practices in the Eurasian Region* (pp. 1–16). IGI Global. https://doi.org/10.4018/978-1-7998-2551-7.ch001

Kumari, S., Patil, Y., & Rao, P. (2017). An Approach to Sustainable Watershed Management: Case Studies on Enhancing Sustainability with Challenges of Water in Western Maharashtra. In P. Rao & Y. Patil (Eds.), *Reconsidering the Impact of Climate Change on Global Water Supply, Use, and Management* (pp. 252–271). Hershey, PA: IGI Global. doi:10.4018/978-1-5225-1046-8.ch014

Kumburu, N. P., & Pande, V. S. (2018). Decentralization and Local Governance in Tanzania: Theories and Practice on Sustainable Development. In K. Teshager Alemu & M. Abebe Alebachew (Eds.), *Handbook of Research on Sustainable Development and Governance Strategies for Economic Growth in Africa* (pp. 131–148). Hershey, PA: IGI Global. doi:10.4018/978-1-5225-3247-7.ch007

Kunock, A. I. (2017). Boko Haram Insurgency in Cameroon: Role of Mass Media in Conflict Management. In N. Mhiripiri & T. Chari (Eds.), *Media Law, Ethics, and Policy in the Digital Age* (pp. 226–244). Hershey, PA: IGI Global. doi:10.4018/978-1-5225-2095-5.ch013

Kurebwa, J. (2019). Young People-Sensitive and Participatory Governance Approaches: Lessons for the Zimbabwean Government. In J. Kurebwa & O. Dodo (Eds.), *Participation of Young People in Governance Processes in Africa* (pp. 80–99). IGI Global. https://doi.org/10.4018/978-1-5225-9388-1.ch005

Lawrie, A. (2017). The Subnational Region: A Utopia? The Challenge of Governing Through Soft Power. In E. Schoburgh & R. Ryan (Eds.), *Handbook of Research on Sub-National Governance and Development* (pp. 96–115). Hershey, PA: IGI Global. doi:10.4018/978-1-5225-1645-3.ch005

Lentzis, D. (2020). Revisiting the Basics of EU Data Protection Law: On the Material and Territorial Scope of the GDPR. In M. Tzanou (Ed.), *Personal Data Protection and Legal Developments in the European Union* (pp. 19–33). IGI Global. https://doi.org/10.4018/978-1-5225-9489-5.ch002

Leote, F. J., Teixeira, N. M., & Galvão, R. (2021). Entrepreneurship and Unemployment: Government Grants and Challenges in a Pandemic Context. In N. Teixeira, & I. Lisboa (Eds.), *Handbook of Research on Financial Management During Economic Downturn and Recovery* (pp. 20-40). IGI Global. https://doi.org/10.4018/978-1-7998-6643-5.ch002

Lewin, E., & Bick, E. (2017). Introduction: Civil Religion and Nationalism on a Godly-Civil Continuum. In E. Lewin, E. Bick, & D. Naor (Eds.), *Comparative Perspectives on Civil Religion, Nationalism, and Political Influence* (pp. 1–31). Hershey, PA: IGI Global. doi:10.4018/978-1-5225-0516-7.ch001

Luyombya, D. (2018). Management of Records and Archives in Uganda's Public Sector. In P. Ngulube (Ed.), *Handbook of Research on Heritage Management and Preservation* (pp. 275–297). Hershey, PA: IGI Global. doi:10.4018/978-1-5225-3137-1.ch014

Mabe, M., & Ashley, E. A. (2017). The Local Command Structure and How the Library Fits. In *In The Developing Role of Public Libraries in Emergency Management: Emerging Research and Opportunities* (pp. 44–60). Hershey, PA: IGI Global. doi:10.4018/978-1-5225-2196-9.ch004

Macilotti, G. (2020). Online Child Pornography: Conceptual Issues and Law Enforcement Challenges. In A. Balloni & R. Sette (Eds.), *Handbook of Research on Trends and Issues in Crime Prevention, Rehabilitation, and Victim Support* (pp. 226–247). IGI Global. https://doi.org/10.4018/978-1-7998-1286-9.ch013

Maher, C. (2018). Legal Framework, Funding, and Procurement Polices to Accelerate the Growth of the Social Enterprise Ecosystem. In *Influence of Public Policy on Small Social Enterprises: Emerging Research and Opportunities* (pp. 52–83). Hershey, PA: IGI Global. doi:10.4018/978-1-5225-2770-1.ch003

Mahmood, M. (2019). Transformation of Government and Citizen Trust in Government: A Conceptual Model. In A. Molnar (Ed.), *Strategic Management and Innovative Applications of E-Government* (pp. 107–122). IGI Global. https://doi.org/10.4018/978-1-5225-6204-7.ch005

Mahmood, Z. (2021). Cloud Computing Technologies for Connected Digital Government. In Z. Mahmood (Ed.), *Web 2.0 and Cloud Technologies for Implementing Connected Government* (pp. 19–35). IGI Global. https://doi.org/10.4018/978-1-7998-4570-6.ch002

Malik, I., Putera, V. S., & Putra, I. E. (2018). Traditional Leaders in the Reconciliation of Muslim-Christian Conflicts in Moluccas. In A. Campbell (Ed.), *Global Leadership Initiatives for Conflict Resolution and Peacebuilding* (pp. 235–248). Hershey, PA: IGI Global. doi:10.4018/978-1-5225-4993-2.ch011

Martin, S. M. (2017). Transnational Crime and the American Policing System. In M. Dawson, D. Kisku, P. Gupta, J. Sing, & W. Li (Eds.), Developing Next-Generation Countermeasures for Homeland Security Threat Prevention (pp. 72-92). Hershey, PA: IGI Global. https://doi.org/ doi:10.4018/978-1-5225-0703-1.ch004

Mekonnen, G. A., & Kassie, W. A. (2020). Fiscal Decentralization at Local Government of Ethiopia: Theory vs Practices. In S. Chhabra & M. Kumar (Eds.), *Civic Engagement Frameworks and Strategic Leadership Practices for Organization Development* (pp. 171–197). IGI Global. https://doi.org/10.4018/978-1-7998-2372-8.ch008

Mensah, I. K., Luo, C., & Abu-Shanab, E. (2021). Citizen Use of E-Government Services Websites: A Proposed E-Government Adoption Recommendation Model (EGARM). *International Journal of Electronic Government Research, 17*(2), 19–42. https://doi.org/10.4018/IJEGR.2021040102

Mhiripiri, N. A., & Chikakano, J. (2017). Criminal Defamation, the Criminalisation of Expression, Media and Information Dissemination in the Digital Age: A Legal and Ethical Perspective. In N. Mhiripiri & T. Chari (Eds.), *Media Law, Ethics, and Policy in the Digital Age* (pp. 1–24). Hershey, PA: IGI Global. doi:10.4018/978-1-5225-2095-5.ch001

Mishaal, D. A., & Abu-Shanab, E. A. (2017). Utilizing Facebook by the Arab World Governments: The Communication Success Factor. *International Journal of Public Administration in the Digital Age, 4*(3), 53–78. doi:10.4018/IJPADA.2017070105

Morim, A. C., Inácio, H., & Vieira, E. (2018). Internal Control in a Public Hospital: The Case of Financial Services Expenditure Department. In G. Azevedo, J. da Silva Oliveira, R. Marques, & A. Ferreira (Eds.), *Handbook of Research on Modernization and Accountability in Public Sector Management* (pp. 77–102). Hershey, PA: IGI Global. doi:10.4018/978-1-5225-3731-1.ch005

Mupepi, M. G. (2017). Developing Democratic Paradigms to Effectively Manage Business, Government, and Civil Society: The African Spring. In E. Schoburgh & R. Ryan (Eds.), *Handbook of Research on Sub-National Governance and Development* (pp. 432–462). Hershey, PA: IGI Global. doi:10.4018/978-1-5225-1645-3.ch020

Mwakisisya, H. J., Rugeiyamu, R., & Cyprian, S. (2021). Blending Local Government Authorities and Grassroots for Industrial Economy Through Participatory Development Communication in Tanzania. In F. Nafukho & A. Boniface Makulilo (Eds.), *Handbook of Research on Nurturing Industrial Economy for Africa's Development* (pp. 74–98). IGI Global. https://doi.org/10.4018/978-1-7998-6471-4.ch005

Naidoo, V., & Nzimakwe, T. I. (2019). M-Government and Its Application on Public Service Delivery. In R. Abassi & A. Ben Chehida Douss (Eds.), *Security Frameworks in Contemporary Electronic Government* (pp. 1–14). IGI Global. https://doi.org/10.4018/978-1-5225-5984-9.ch001

Navaratnam, R., & Lee, I. Y. (2017). Globalization as a New Framework for Human Rights Protection. In C. Akrivopoulou (Ed.), *Defending Human Rights and Democracy in the Era of Globalization* (pp. 17–49). Hershey, PA: IGI Global. doi:10.4018/978-1-5225-0723-9.ch002

Nemec, J., Meričková, B. M., Svidroňová, M. M., & Klimovský, D. (2017). Co-Creation as a Social Innovation in Delivery of Public Services at Local Government Level: The Slovak Experience. In E. Schoburgh & R. Ryan (Eds.), *Handbook of Research on Sub-National Governance and Development* (pp. 281–303). Hershey, PA: IGI Global. doi:10.4018/978-1-5225-1645-3.ch013

Neupane, A., Soar, J., Vaidya, K., & Aryal, S. (2017). Application of E-Government Principles in Anti-Corruption Framework. In R. Shakya (Ed.), *Digital Governance and E-Government Principles Applied to Public Procurement* (pp. 56–74). Hershey, PA: IGI Global. doi:10.4018/978-1-5225-2203-4.ch003

Njie, S. N., Wogu, I. A., Ogbuehi, U. K., Misra, S., & Udoh, O. D. (2021). Rising Global Challenges in Energy Demand and the Politics of Climate Change in Government Operations: Policy and Economic Development Implications. In C. Babaoğlu, E. Akman, & O. Kulaç (Eds.), *Handbook of Research on Global Challenges for Improving Public Services and Government Operations* (pp. 242–263). IGI Global. https://doi.org/10.4018/978-1-7998-4978-0.ch013

Ogunde, O. (2017). Democracy and Child Rights Protection: The Problem of the Nigerian Constitution. In C. Akrivopoulou (Ed.), *Defending Human Rights and Democracy in the Era of Globalization* (pp. 123–144). Hershey, PA: IGI Global. doi:10.4018/978-1-5225-0723-9.ch006

Ojedokun, U. A. (2017). Crime Witnesses' Non-Cooperation in Police Investigations: Causes and Consequences in Nigeria. In S. Egharevba (Ed.), *Police Brutality, Racial Profiling, and Discrimination in the Criminal Justice System* (pp. 89–99). Hershey, PA: IGI Global. doi:10.4018/978-1-5225-1088-8.ch005

Okeke, G. S. (2018). The Politics of Environmental Pollution in Nigeria: Emerging Trends, Issues, and Challenges. In A. Eneanya (Ed.), *Handbook of Research on Environmental Policies for Emergency Management and Public Safety* (pp. 300–320). Hershey, PA: IGI Global. doi:10.4018/978-1-5225-3194-4.ch016

Ökten, S., Akman, E., & Akman, Ç. (2018). Modernization and Accountability in Public-Sector Administration: Turkey Example. In G. Azevedo, J. da Silva Oliveira, R. Marques, & A. Ferreira (Eds.), *Handbook of Research on Modernization and Accountability in Public Sector Management* (pp. 18–39). Hershey, PA: IGI Global. doi:10.4018/978-1-5225-3731-1.ch002

Oladapo, O. A., & Ojebuyi, B. R. (2017). Nature and Outcome of Nigeria's #NoToSocialMediaBill Twitter Protest against the Frivolous Petitions Bill 2015. In O. Nelson, B. Ojebuyi, & A. Salawu (Eds.), *Impacts of the Media on African Socio-Economic Development* (pp. 106–124). Hershey, PA: IGI Global. doi:10.4018/978-1-5225-1859-4.ch007

Olmos, S., & Nares, J. J. (2020). Applying Fault Trees to the Analysis at the Minimum Age for Sexual Consent in the Criminal Law of México. In A. Balloni & R. Sette (Eds.), *Handbook of Research on Trends and Issues in Crime Prevention, Rehabilitation, and Victim Support* (pp. 60–78). IGI Global. https://doi.org/10.4018/978-1-7998-1286-9.ch005

Olukolu, Y. R. (2017). Harmful Traditional Practices, Laws, and Reproductive Rights of Women in Nigeria: A Therapeutic Jurisprudence Approach. In D. Halder & K. Jaishankar (Eds.), *Therapeutic Jurisprudence and Overcoming Violence Against Women* (pp. 1–14). Hershey, PA: IGI Global. doi:10.4018/978-1-5225-2472-4.ch001

Onyebadi, U., & Mbunyuza-Memani, L. (2017). Women and South Africa's Anti-Apartheid Struggle: Evaluating the Political Messages in the Music of Miriam Makeba. In U. Onyebadi (Ed.), *Music as a Platform for Political Communication* (pp. 31–51). Hershey, PA: IGI Global. doi:10.4018/978-1-5225-1986-7.ch002

Osmani, A. R. (2017). Tipaimukh Multipurpose Hydroelectric Project: A Policy Perspective – Indo-Bangla Priorities, Indigenous Peoples' Rights, and Environmental Concerns. In P. Rao & Y. Patil (Eds.), *Reconsidering the Impact of Climate Change on Global Water Supply, Use, and Management* (pp. 227–251). Hershey, PA: IGI Global. doi:10.4018/978-1-5225-1046-8.ch013

Owolabi, T. O. (2018). Free Media and Bank Reforms in West Africa: Implications for Sustainable Development. In A. Salawu & T. Owolabi (Eds.), *Exploring Journalism Practice and Perception in Developing Countries* (pp. 18–39). Hershey, PA: IGI Global. doi:10.4018/978-1-5225-3376-4.ch002

Öztürk, N. K. (2021). Government Systems and Control of Bureaucracy. In C. Babaoğlu, E. Akman, & O. Kulaç (Eds.), *Handbook of Research on Global Challenges for Improving Public Services and Government Operations* (pp. 133–150). IGI Global. https://doi.org/10.4018/978-1-7998-4978-0.ch008

Pacheco, F. M., & Alves, D. R. (2019). The New Paths of Fundamental Rights in the 21st Century: Globalization and Knowledge in a Digital Age as a Proposal. In A. Melro & L. Oliveira (Eds.), *Constitutional Knowledge and Its Impact on Citizenship Exercise in a Networked Society* (pp. 1–26). IGI Global. https://doi.org/10.4018/978-1-5225-8350-9.ch001

Panda, P., & Sahu, G. P. (2017). Public Procurement Framework in India: An Overview. In R. Shakya (Ed.), *Digital Governance and E-Government Principles Applied to Public Procurement* (pp. 229–248). Hershey, PA: IGI Global. doi:10.4018/978-1-5225-2203-4.ch010

Pande, V. S., & Kumburu, N. P. (2018). An Overview of Population Growth and Sustainable Development in Sub-Saharan Africa. In K. Teshager Alemu & M. Abebe Alebachew (Eds.), *Handbook of Research on Sustainable Development and Governance Strategies for Economic Growth in Africa* (pp. 480–499). Hershey, PA: IGI Global. doi:10.4018/978-1-5225-3247-7.ch025

Parikh, M., & Krishna, V. S. (2021). Recent Trends and Repercussions in Civil and Criminal Justice Systems: A Comparative Analysis of England, Singapore, and India. In E. Yin, & N. Kofie (Ed.), *Advancing Civil Justice Reform and Conflict Resolution in Africa and Asia: Comparative Analyses and Case Studies* (pp. 230-242). IGI Global. https://doi.org/10.4018/978-1-7998-7898-8.ch013

Pattnaik, P. N., & Shukla, M. K. (2020). Understanding Indian Political Parties Through the Lens of Marketing Management: Towards a Conceptual Political Marketing Model. In S. Kavoğlu & M. Salar (Eds.), *Political Propaganda, Advertising, and Public Relations: Emerging Research and Opportunities* (pp. 170–190). IGI Global. https://doi.org/10.4018/978-1-7998-1734-5.ch008

Paulin, A. A. (2017). Informating Public Governance: Towards a Basis for a Digital Ecosystem. *International Journal of Public Administration in the Digital Age*, *4*(2), 14–32. doi:10.4018/IJPADA.2017040102

Perelló-Sobrepere, M. (2017). Building a New State from Outrage: The Case of Catalonia. In M. Adria & Y. Mao (Eds.), *Handbook of Research on Citizen Engagement and Public Participation in the Era of New Media* (pp. 344–359). Hershey, PA: IGI Global. doi:10.4018/978-1-5225-1081-9.ch019

Pohl, G. M. (2017). The Role of Social Media in Enforcing Environmental Justice around the World. In K. Demirhan & D. Çakır-Demirhan (Eds.), *Political Scandal, Corruption, and Legitimacy in the Age of Social Media* (pp. 123–156). Hershey, PA: IGI Global. doi:10.4018/978-1-5225-2019-1.ch006

Popescu, C. R. (2022). Environmental, Social, and Corporate Governance by Avoiding Management Bias and Tax Minimization: Reaching a General Consensus Regarding a Minimum Global Tax Rate. In C. Popescu (Ed.), *COVID-19 Pandemic Impact on New Economy Development and Societal Change* (pp. 94–132). IGI Global. https://doi.org/10.4018/978-1-6684-3374-4.ch006

Popoola, T. (2017). Ethical and Legal Challenges of Election Reporting in Nigeria: A Study of Four General Elections, 1999-2011. In N. Mhiripiri & T. Chari (Eds.), *Media Law, Ethics, and Policy in the Digital Age* (pp. 78–100). Hershey, PA: IGI Global. doi:10.4018/978-1-5225-2095-5.ch005

Prakash, O. (2020). History, Policy Making, and Sustainability. In R. Das & N. Mandal (Eds.), *Interdisciplinary Approaches to Public Policy and Sustainability* (pp. 1–17). IGI Global. https://doi.org/10.4018/978-1-7998-0315-7.ch001

Provazníková, R., Sobotková, L., & Sobotka, M. (2021). Local Government Development in the Czech Republic: Dilemmas and Challenges. In C. Babaoğlu, E. Akman, & O. Kulaç (Eds.), *Handbook of Research on Global Challenges for Improving Public Services and Government Operations* (pp. 151–171). IGI Global. https://doi.org/10.4018/978-1-7998-4978-0.ch009

Qawasmeh, F. A. (2022). Understanding the Field of Public Policy in the Context of Public Administration Evolution. In O. Kulaç, C. Babaoğlu, & E. Akman (Eds.), *Public Affairs Education and Training in the 21st Century* (pp. 22–44). IGI Global. https://doi.org/10.4018/978-1-7998-8243-5.ch002

Rahman, M. S. (2017). Politics-Administration Relations and the Effect on Local Governance and Development: The Case of Bangladesh. In E. Schoburgh & R. Ryan (Eds.), *Handbook of Research on Sub-National Governance and Development* (pp. 256–279). Hershey, PA: IGI Global. doi:10.4018/978-1-5225-1645-3.ch012

Ramachandran, M., Chelliah, P. R., & Soundarabai, P. B. (2021). Towards Connected Government Services: A Cloud Software Engineering Framework. In Z. Mahmood (Ed.), *Web 2.0 and Cloud Technologies for Implementing Connected Government* (pp. 113–135). IGI Global. https://doi.org/10.4018/978-1-7998-4570-6.ch006

Ravotti, N. (2020). In the [Source] C\ode of the Conquerors: On the Need for Culturally-Minded Tribal Law Research Databases. In S. Edwards III, & D. Santos (Eds.), *Digital Transformation and Its Role in Progressing the Relationship Between States and Their Citizens* (pp. 124-137). IGI Global. https://doi.org/10.4018/978-1-7998-3152-5.ch006

Razzante, R. (2020). The Fight Against Corruption. In A. Balloni & R. Sette (Eds.), *Handbook of Research on Trends and Issues in Crime Prevention, Rehabilitation, and Victim Support* (pp. 167–186). IGI Global. doi:10.4018/978-1-7998-1286-9.ch010

Reddy, P. S. (2017). Political-Administrative Interface at the Local Sphere of Government with Particular Reference to South Africa. In E. Schoburgh & R. Ryan (Eds.), *Handbook of Research on Sub-National Governance and Development* (pp. 242–255). Hershey, PA: IGI Global. doi:10.4018/978-1-5225-1645-3.ch011

Rombo, D. O., & Lutomia, A. N. (2018). Tracing the Rights of Domestic and International Kenyan House Helps: Profiles, Policy, and Consequences. In N. Mahtab, T. Haque, I. Khan, M. Islam, & I. Wahid (Eds.), *Handbook of Research on Women's Issues and Rights in the Developing World* (pp. 1–18). Hershey, PA: IGI Global. doi:10.4018/978-1-5225-3018-3.ch001

Rouzbehani, K. (2017). Health Policy Implementation: Moving Beyond Its Barriers in United States. In N. Wickramasinghe (Ed.), *Handbook of Research on Healthcare Administration and Management* (pp. 541–552). Hershey, PA: IGI Global. doi:10.4018/978-1-5225-0920-2.ch032

Ryan, R., & Woods, R. (2017). Decentralization and Subnational Governance: Theory and Praxis. In E. Schoburgh & R. Ryan (Eds.), *Handbook of Research on Sub-National Governance and Development* (pp. 1–33). Hershey, PA: IGI Global. doi:10.4018/978-1-5225-1645-3.ch001

Sabao, C., & Chingwaramusee, V. R. (2017). Citizen Journalism on Facebook and the Challenges of Media Regulation in Zimbabwe: Baba Jukwa. In N. Mhiripiri & T. Chari (Eds.), *Media Law, Ethics, and Policy in the Digital Age* (pp. 193–206). Hershey, PA: IGI Global. doi:10.4018/978-1-5225-2095-5.ch011

Saidane, A., & Al-Sharieh, S. (2019). A Compliance-Driven Framework for Privacy and Security in Highly Regulated Socio-Technical Environments: An E-Government Case Study. In R. Abassi & A. Ben Chehida Douss (Eds.), *Security Frameworks in Contemporary Electronic Government* (pp. 15–50). IGI Global. https://doi.org/10.4018/978-1-5225-5984-9.ch002

Sandill, S. (2020). Law, Equality, and Entrepreneurship Through a Gendered Lens: Bridging the Gap Between Academia, Legislature, and Politics. In T. Moeke-Pickering, S. Cote-Meek, & A. Pegoraro (Eds.), *Critical Reflections and Politics on Advancing Women in the Academy* (pp. 124–149). IGI Global. https://doi.org/10.4018/978-1-7998-3618-6.ch008

Santos, H. R., & Tonelli, D. F. (2019). Smart Government and the Maturity Levels of Sociopolitical Digital Interactions: Analysing Temporal Changes in Brazilian E-Government Portals. In A. Molnar (Ed.), *Strategic Management and Innovative Applications of E-Government* (pp. 176–199). IGI Global. https://doi.org/10.4018/978-1-5225-6204-7.ch008

Saponaro, A. (2021). "Visible" and "Invisible" Victims in the Criminal Justice System: Victim-Oriented Paradigms and Models. In R. Blasdell, L. Krieger-Sample, & M. Kilburn (Eds.), *Invisible Victims and the Pursuit of Justice: Analyzing Frequently Victimized Yet Rarely Discussed Populations* (pp. 1–23). IGI Global. doi:10.4018/978-1-7998-7348-8.ch001

Shaikh, A. K., Ahmad, N., Khan, I., & Ali, S. (2021). E-Participation Within E-Government: A Bibliometric-Based Systematic Literature Review. *International Journal of Electronic Government Research*, *17*(4), 15–39. https://doi.org/10.4018/IJEGR.2021100102

Shakya, R. K., & Schapper, P. R. (2017). Digital Governance and E-Government Principles: E-Procurement as Transformative. In R. Shakya (Ed.), *Digital Governance and E-Government Principles Applied to Public Procurement* (pp. 1–28). Hershey, PA: IGI Global. doi:10.4018/978-1-5225-2203-4.ch001

Shambare, R. (2019). Facilitating Consumers' Adoption of E-Government in South Africa: Supply Side-Driven Virtuous Cycles. In A. Gbadamosi (Ed.), *Exploring the Dynamics of Consumerism in Developing Nations* (pp. 243–265). IGI Global. https://doi.org/10.4018/978-1-5225-7906-9.ch011

Siphambe, H., Kolobe, M., & Oageng, I. P. (2018). Employment Protection Legislation and Unemployment in Botswana. In S. Amine (Ed.), *Employment Protection Legislation in Emerging Economies* (pp. 157–191). Hershey, PA: IGI Global. doi:10.4018/978-1-5225-4134-9.ch008

Song, M. Y., & Abelson, J. (2017). Public Engagement and Policy Entrepreneurship on Social Media in the Time of Anti-Vaccination Movements. In M. Adria & Y. Mao (Eds.), *Handbook of Research on Citizen Engagement and Public Participation in the Era of New Media* (pp. 38–56). Hershey, PA: IGI Global. doi:10.4018/978-1-5225-1081-9.ch003

Sood, P., Malhotra, M., & Nijjer, S. (2021). Government Policies During Lockdown: Indian vs. International Perspective. In V. Kumar & G. Malhotra (Eds.), *Stakeholder Strategies for Reducing the Impact of Global Health Crises* (pp. 18–39). IGI Global. https://doi.org/10.4018/978-1-7998-7495-9.ch002

Stacey, E. (2018). Networked Protests: A Review of Social Movement Literature and the Hong Kong Umbrella Movement (2017). In S. Chhabra (Ed.), *Handbook of Research on Civic Engagement and Social Change in Contemporary Society* (pp. 347–363). Hershey, PA: IGI Global. doi:10.4018/978-1-5225-4197-4.ch020

Stamatakis, N. (2017). Authority and Legitimacy: A Quantitative Study of Youth's Perceptions on the Brazilian Police. In S. Egharevba (Ed.), *Police Brutality, Racial Profiling, and Discrimination in the Criminal Justice System* (pp. 151–213). Hershey, PA: IGI Global. doi:10.4018/978-1-5225-1088-8.ch009

Steinert, S. W. (2021). An Interview With Chief Sargent of the Worcester, MA Police Department. In E. Arble & B. Arnetz (Eds.), *Interventions, Training, and Technologies for Improved Police Well-Being and Performance* (pp. 185–197). IGI Global. https://doi.org/10.4018/978-1-7998-6820-0.ch011

Sugars, J. M. (2017). Refoulement and Refugees. In C. Akrivopoulou (Ed.), *Defending Human Rights and Democracy in the Era of Globalization* (pp. 181–197). Hershey, PA: IGI Global. doi:10.4018/978-1-5225-0723-9.ch008

Takaya-Umehara, Y. (2019). Suborbital Spaceflight: Legal Aspects. In A. Nakarada Pecujlic & M. Tugnoli (Eds.), *Promoting Productive Cooperation Between Space Lawyers and Engineers* (pp. 64–78). IGI Global. https://doi.org/10.4018/978-1-5225-7256-5.ch005

Tan, S. F. (2017). Local Representation in Australia: Preliminary Findings of a National Survey. In E. Schoburgh & R. Ryan (Eds.), *Handbook of Research on Sub-National Governance and Development* (pp. 368–384). Hershey, PA: IGI Global. doi:10.4018/978-1-5225-1645-3.ch017

Tavares, M. D., & Rodrigues, L. L. (2018). Strategic Responses of Public Sector Entities to GRI Sustainability Reports. In G. Azevedo, J. da Silva Oliveira, R. Marques, & A. Ferreira (Eds.), *Handbook of Research on Modernization and Accountability in Public Sector Management* (pp. 159–188). Hershey, PA: IGI Global. doi:10.4018/978-1-5225-3731-1.ch008

Thakre, A. G. (2017). Sexual Harassment of Women in Workplace in India: An Assessment of Implementation of Preventive Laws and Practicing of Therapeutic Jurisprudence in New Delhi. In D. Halder & K. Jaishankar (Eds.), *Therapeutic Jurisprudence and Overcoming Violence Against Women* (pp. 135–146). Hershey, PA: IGI Global. doi:10.4018/978-1-5225-2472-4.ch009

Tiwary, A. (2017). Key Elements of CEAF. In *Driving Efficiency in Local Government Using a Collaborative Enterprise Architecture Framework: Emerging Research and Opportunities* (pp. 25–61). Hershey, PA: IGI Global. doi:10.4018/978-1-5225-2407-6.ch002

Toscano, J. P. (2017). Social Media and Public Participation: Opportunities, Barriers, and a New Framework. In M. Adria & Y. Mao (Eds.), *Handbook of Research on Citizen Engagement and Public Participation in the Era of New Media* (pp. 73–89). Hershey, PA: IGI Global. doi:10.4018/978-1-5225-1081-9.ch005

Trompetter, P. S. (2019). A History of Police Psychology. In I. Management Association (Eds.), *Police Science: Breakthroughs in Research and Practice* (pp. 377-402). IGI Global. https://doi.org/10.4018/978-1-5225-7672-3.ch019

Tryma, K., & Salnikova, N. (2021). The Influence of Religion on Political Parties of the European Union. In E. Alaverdov & M. Bari (Eds.), *Global Development of Religious Tourism* (pp. 98-112). IGI Global. https://doi.org/10.4018/978-1-7998-5792-1.ch007

Tsabedze, V. W. (2020). Strategies for Managing E-Records for Good Governance: Reflection on E-Government in the Kingdom of Eswatini. In M. Rodríguez Bolívar & M. Cortés Cediel (Eds.), *Digital Government and Achieving E-Public Participation: Emerging Research and Opportunities* (pp. 63–86). IGI Global. https://doi.org/10.4018/978-1-7998-1526-6.ch004

Tshishonga, N. (2017). Operation Sukuma-Sakhe: A New Social Contract for Decentralized Service Delivery and Responsive Governance in KwaZulu-Natal. In E. Schoburgh & R. Ryan (Eds.), *Handbook of Research on Sub-National Governance and Development* (pp. 304–323). Hershey, PA: IGI Global. doi:10.4018/978-1-5225-1645-3.ch014

Tsygankov, S., & Gasanova, E. (2017). Electronification of the Public Procurement System: A Comparative Analysis of the Experience of the Russian Federation and Ukraine. In R. Shakya (Ed.), *Digital Governance and E-Government Principles Applied to Public Procurement* (pp. 267–277). Hershey, PA: IGI Global. doi:10.4018/978-1-5225-2203-4.ch013

Tüzünkan, D. (2018). The International Migration Movements and Immigrant Policies From the Ottoman Empire 1299 to Republican Turkey 2016. In Ş. Erçetin (Ed.), *Social Considerations of Migration Movements and Immigration Policies* (pp. 13–45). Hershey, PA: IGI Global. doi:10.4018/978-1-5225-3322-1.ch002

Ullah, Z. (2022). Violent Extremism and the Politics of Education in Pakistan: An Analysis of the Links Between Anti-Terror Laws, the Curriculum, and the Islamised Public Sphere. In O. Kulaç, C. Babaoğlu, & E. Akman (Eds.), *Public Affairs Education and Training in the 21st Century* (pp. 256–275). IGI Global. https://doi.org/10.4018/978-1-7998-8243-5.ch017

Valenzuela, R., & Ochoa, A. (2018). Open Mexico Network in the Implementation of National Open Data Policy. In A. Kok (Ed.), *Proliferation of Open Government Initiatives and Systems* (pp. 50–67). Hershey, PA: IGI Global. doi:10.4018/978-1-5225-4987-1.ch003

Valera-Ordaz, L., & Humanes, M. L. (2022). What Drives Selective Exposure to Political Information in Spain? Comparing Political Interest and Ideology. In D. Palau-Sampio, G. López García, & L. Iannelli (Eds.), *Contemporary Politics, Communication, and the Impact on Democracy* (pp. 93–112). IGI Global. https://doi.org/10.4018/978-1-7998-8057-8.ch006

van der Vliet-Bakker, J. M. (2019). Environmentally Forced Migration and Human Rights. In I. Management Association (Eds.), *Immigration and Refugee Policy: Breakthroughs in Research and Practice* (pp. 336-362). IGI Global. https://doi.org/10.4018/978-1-5225-8909-9.ch019

Waller, P. (2017). Co-Production and Co-Creation in Public Services: Resolving Confusion and Contradictions. *International Journal of Electronic Government Research, 13*(2), 1–17. doi:10.4018/IJEGR.2017040101

Wodecka-Hyjek, A. (2017). Co-Operation between the Public Administration and Non-Profit Organisations as a Condition of the Development of Public Entrepreneurship: On the Example of the Selected World Solutions. In V. Potocan, M. Ünğan, & Z. Nedelko (Eds.), *Handbook of Research on Managerial Solutions in Non-Profit Organizations* (pp. 253–275). Hershey, PA: IGI Global. doi:10.4018/978-1-5225-0731-4.ch012

Yang, K. C., & Kang, Y. (2017). Social Media, Political Mobilization, and Citizen Engagement: A Case Study of the March 18, 2014, Sunflower Student Movement in Taiwan. In M. Adria & Y. Mao (Eds.), *Handbook of Research on Citizen Engagement and Public Participation in the Era of New Media* (pp. 360–388). Hershey, PA: IGI Global. doi:10.4018/978-1-5225-1081-9.ch020

Yang, K. C., & Kang, Y. (2020). Will Microblogs Shape China's Civil Society Under President's Xi's Surveillance State?: The Case of Anti-Extradition Law Protests in Hong Kong. In V. Kumar & G. Malhotra (Eds.), *Examining the Roles of IT and Social Media in Democratic Development and Social Change* (pp. 156–184). IGI Global. https://doi.org/10.4018/978-1-7998-1791-8.ch007

Yasmeen, H., Wang, Y., Zameer, H., & Ismail, H. (2020). Modeling the Role of Government, Firm, and Civil Society for Environmental Sustainability. In I. Management Association (Ed.), *Developing Eco-Cities Through Policy, Planning, and Innovation: Can It Really Work?* (pp. 62-83). IGI Global. https://doi.org/10.4018/978-1-7998-0441-3.ch003

Yavuz, N., Karkın, N., & Sevinç Çubuk, E. B. (2020). Explaining Government Crowdsourcing Decisions: A Theoretical Model. In M. Rodríguez Bolívar & M. Cortés Cediel (Eds.), *Digital Government and Achieving E-Public Participation: Emerging Research and Opportunities* (pp. 159–183). IGI Global. https://doi.org/10.4018/978-1-7998-1526-6.ch008

Zhaleleva, S., Zhaleleva, R., & Pasternak, A. (2020). Evolution of Business-Government Interaction Models: Their Use and Management. In G. Tazhina & J. Parker (Eds.), *Toward Sustainability Through Digital Technologies and Practices in the Eurasian Region* (pp. 17–35). IGI Global. https://doi.org/10.4018/978-1-7998-2551-7.ch002

Zhao, B. (2018). A Privacy Perspective of Open Government: Sex, Wealth, and Transparency in China. In A. Kok (Ed.), *Proliferation of Open Government Initiatives and Systems* (pp. 29–48). Hershey, PA: IGI Global. doi:10.4018/978-1-5225-4987-1.ch002

About the Contributors

Nikolaos Karagiannis is a Research Scholar at the Global Institute for Sustainable Prosperity, a Professor of Economics at Winston-Salem State University, North Carolina, an invited visiting scholar at the University of Cambridge, England; and the co-editor of American Review of Political Economy. He has published extensively in the areas of economic development, public sector economics, and macroeconomic policy analysis. Professor Karagiannis is particularly interested in developmental state theory and policy, and his research has focused on the applicability of this perspective in different contexts such as in EU countries, the United States, Caribbean small island economies, North African countries, and China. He is the author, co-author and co-editor of twenty three books and has published over 160 papers as refereed journal articles, book chapters and op-eds.

Sheilia Goodwin is an Assistant Professor of Community Health Nursing and Research at Winston-Salem State University, North Carolina. She has co-authored several research articles, and has collaborated in projects and proposals in the areas of Community Health administration and policy. She is an active member of various organizations related to her areas of expertise.

David Stewart is an Associate Professor of Finance at Winston-Salem State University, North Carolina. He has co-authored several research articles and a textbook. His interest in United States healthcare stems from his primary research area of personal financial planning.

Melissa R. Bowman Foster is an Associate Professor in the School of Health Sciences at Winston-Salem State University and currently teaches at both the undergraduate and graduate levels. She also serves as the Program Coordinator for the Master of Health Administration program. She has over two decades of experience in the health care field that encompasses the areas of radiology, medical assisting, phlebotomy, nursing, EKG, research, medical billing & coding, pathology, 3D image processing, and clinical education. She is also a published scholar and member of the American Society for Radiologic Technologists, an advocate for the CARE Bill for NCSRT, and a motivational speaker for working parents. Her research interests include radiology education, phlebotomy training practices, COVID-19 research, infectious disease control, infectious disease treatment, and competency based education .

Aparna A. Gosavi is an Associate Professor of Finance in Winston-Salem State University. Her research interests are in corporate finance and economic development. She has a PhD and an MS in Finance. Her BS degree is in Electronics. Her research has appeared in prominent journals of her field, e.g., Journal of African Business and the International Trade Journal.

Abhijit Gosavi is an Associate Professor of Engineering Management and Systems Engineering at Missouri University of Science and Technology at Rolla, MO, USA. His research interests are simulation-based optimization, Markov decision processes, and production management. He is the author of the Springer text Simulation-Based Optimization: Parametric Optimization Techniques and Reinforcement Learning, now in its second edition. He has a BS and an MTech in Mechanical Engineering and a PhD in industrial engineering.

Benjamin Greene served as the Practice Administrator of Cornerstone Hematology/Oncology in High Point, NC, co-authoring the only approved CMS Innovation Center Oncology Care Model grant in North Carolina. Previously, he worked in the Office of the Dean at the School of Business and Economics at Winston-Salem State University (WSSU) and served as Executive Director/CEO of U.S. symphony orchestras. He has a Master's in Healthcare Administration from WSSU and a Master's in Arts Administration from Indiana University. He served the National Endowment for the Arts, the Florida and California Arts Councils as a grants review panelist, and chaired national and statewide conference seminars in labor relations and orchestra management. He was President of the Florida Association of Symphony Orchestras, Treasurer of the Association of California Symphony Orchestras; and co-authored journal articles on Computer Self-Efficacy and Facilitating Conditions on Student Computer Use.

Jill Harp, Ph.D. is Interim Director of the Biomedical Research Infrastructure Center, and Professor of Biochemistry in the departments of Biological Sciences and Chemistry at Winston-Salem State University (WSSU) and an Adjunct Professor at Wake Forest University Health Sciences (WFUHS) in the Physiology and Pharmacology Department. She received her BS degree from the York College-City University of New York and her Ph.D. from the University of Maryland-College

Park. Dr. Harp teaches nursing chemistry, biology, ad chemistry courses. She is a bioorganic chemist with training in pharmacology and conducts research related to CNS disease/disorders. Dr. Harp is involved in the assessment of student learning, served on various Accreditation Leadership Teams and Assessment Committees, has served as chair of the Quality Enhancement Plan (QEP) Topics Selection Committee, co-chaired the QEP Development Committee, and served as a co-chair of the QEP Steering Committee. In 2011, Dr. Harp received the Board of Governors award for Excellence in Teaching. Faculty development is important to Dr. Harp and collaborative activities have led to several conference presentations in writing, critical thinking, curriculum enhancements, and faculty development, to name a few. Dr. Harp is also involved with outreach activities involving K12 youth. She is one of the founders of SciTech which incorporates performing hands-on experiments with elementary through high school-aged students.

Stephanie E Joseph is a co-chair and associate professor in the Department of Healthcare Management of the School of Health Sciences at Winston-Salem State University (WSSU), and an attorney licensed to practice law in California and Michigan. She was a pre-law student at Appalachian State University where she earned a BS in Sociology, with a concentration in legal studies and a minor in criminal justice. She received her JD from Pepperdine University School of Law in 2000 and began her professional career in the law firm setting where she represented clients primarily in the areas of business management, human resources, premises liability, medical malpractice, and associated personal injury matters. She joined the faculty of WSSU in 2006, where she teaches classes and creates curriculum at the undergraduate and graduate levels. Her particular emphasis is in law, ethics, and policy in managerial decision-making and business technology.

Yifei Liu is an Associate Professor at the University of Missouri-Kansas City (UMKC) School of Pharmacy; a fellow at UMKC Healthcare Institute for Innovations in Quality; and a doctoral faculty member at UMKC Henry W. Bloch School of Management. He has a B.S. in Pharmacy from West China University of Medical Sciences, and an M.S. and a Ph.D. in Pharmaceutical Socioeconomics from University of Iowa. Liu has taught a multitude of topics in the areas of the U.S. healthcare system, healthcare marketing, pharmacy practice management, health economics, and healthcare policy. He has extensive research experience in implementing and evaluating healthcare services, examining the behaviors of patients or healthcare professionals, and identifying factors impacting healthcare utilization. His research has been funded by government agencies, professional organizations, and pharmaceutical manufacturers.

Zagros Madjd-Sadjadi is Full Professor of Economics at Winston-Salem State University, the Department Chair for Accounting, Economics, and Finance, and a Research Fellow of the Center for the Study of Economic Mobility.

Enrico Marcelli is Associate Professor of Sociology at San Diego State University. He has held several NIH grants, has authored several publications in the area of health economics and policy, and was a Robert Wood Johnson Scholar at Harvard University .

C.J. Polychroniou is a political scientist/political economist, author, and journalist who has taught and worked in numerous universities and research centers in Europe and the United States. Currently, his main research interests are in U.S. politics and the political economy of the United States, European economic integration, globalization, climate change and environmental economics, and the deconstruction of neoliberalism's politico-economic project. Polychroniou is a regular contributor to Truthout as well as a member of Truthout's Public Intellectual Project. He has published scores of books and over 1,000 articles which have appeared in a variety of journals, magazines, newspapers, and popular news websites. Many of his publications have been translated into a multitude of different languages, including Arabic, Chinese, Croatian, Dutch, French, German, Greek, Italian, Japanese, Portuguese, Russian, Spanish and Turkish.

Darryl Scriven is a graduate of both Florida A&M University and Purdue University with degrees in Mathematics and Philosophy. He was a Fulbright Scholar to Morocco and Tunisia, and has taught at Wilberforce University, Southern University-Baton Rouge, and at the Tuskegee University National Center for Bioethics in Research and Health Care. Dr. Scriven was Dean of the College of Arts, Sciences, Business and Education as well as the John and Anna Hanes Distinguished Professor in the Humanities at Winston-Salem State University. He is currently Dean of Arts and Sciences at Clarkson University and serves as Academic Chair of the Journal of Science, Healthcare, and the Humanities.

Martha Tepepa was born and raised in Mexico City. She holds a PhD from El Colegio de Mexico and an M.A. from Columbia University. Her academic research uses a multidisciplinary approach to analyze the power structures and economic obstacles that prevent urban and rural communities to achieve a dignified life. Tepepa has examined various social policies implemented in Latin American from a gender, environmental, and social justice perspective. Her extensive fieldwork conducted in popular neighborhoods in the province of Buenos Aires, Argentina has allowed her to observe the effects of economic crises in the lives of people that inhabit irregular settlements with environmental and health hazards, and high rates of crime and unemployment. Her background in economics has allowed her to transform ethnographic data into a multidimensional poverty index. Dr Tepepa believes in the power of multiculturalism to gain new insights and to show new directions for knowledge and understanding of each other.

Index

W

www.ingramcontent.com/pod-product-compliance
Lightning Source LLC
LaVergne TN
LVHW061536290926
849162LV00004B/808
* 9 7 8 1 6 6 8 4 4 0 6 0 5 *